For the Record

Protecting Electronic Health Information

Committee on Maintaining Privacy and Security in
Health Care Applications of the
National Information Infrastructure

Computer Science and Telecommunications Board
Commission on Physical Sciences, Mathematics, and Applications
National Research Council

NATIONAL ACADEMY PRESS
Washington, D.C. 1997

NOTICE: The project that is the subject of this report was approved by the Governing Board of the National Research Council, whose members are drawn from the councils of the National Academy of Sciences, the National Academy of Engineering, and the Institute of Medicine. The members of the committee responsible for the report were chosen for their special competences and with regard for appropriate balance.

This report has been reviewed by a group other than the authors according to procedures approved by a Report Review Committee consisting of members of the National Academy of Sciences, the National Academy of Engineering, and the Institute of Medicine.

Support for this project was provided by the National Library of Medicine and the Warren Grant Magnuson Clinical Center of the National Institutes of Health and by the Massachusetts Health Data Consortium. Any opinions, findings, conclusions, or recommendations expressed in this material are those of the authors and do not necessarily reflect the views of the sponsors.

Library of Congress Catalog Card Number 97-65240
International Standard Book Number 0-309-05697-7

Additional copies of this report are available from:

National Academy Press
2101 Constitution Avenue, NW
Box 285
Washington, DC 20055
800/624-6242
202/334-3313 (in the Washington Metropolitan Area)
http://www.nap.edu

iii

The National Academy of Sciences is a private, nonprofit, self-perpetuating society of distinguished scholars engaged in scientific and engineering research, dedicated to the furtherance of science and technology and to their use for the general welfare. Upon the authority of the charter granted to it by the Congress in 1863, the Academy has a mandate that requires it to advise the federal government on scientific and technical matters. Dr. Bruce Alberts is president of the National Academy of Sciences.

The National Academy of Engineering was established in 1964, under the charter of the National Academy of Sciences, as a parallel organization of outstanding engineers. It is autonomous in its administration and in the selection of its members, sharing with the National Academy of Sciences the responsibility for advising the federal government. The National Academy of Engineering also sponsors engineering programs aimed at meeting national needs, encourages education and research, and recognizes the superior achievements of engineers. Dr. William A. Wulf is president of the National Academy of Engineering.

The Institute of Medicine was established in 1970 by the National Academy of Sciences to secure the services of eminent members of appropriate professions in the examination of policy matters pertaining to the health of the public. The Institute acts under the responsibility given to the National Academy of Sciences by its congressional charter to be an adviser to the federal government and, upon its own initiative, to identify issues of medical care, research, and education. Dr. Kenneth I. Shine is president of the Institute of Medicine.

The National Research Council was organized by the National Academy of Sciences in 1916 to associate the broad community of science and technology with the Academy's purposes of furthering knowledge and advising the federal government. Functioning in accordance with general policies determined by the Academy, the Council has become the principal operating agency of both the National Academy of Sciences and the National Academy of Engineering in providing services to the government, the public, and the scientific and engineering communities. The Council is administered jointly by both Academies and the Institute of Medicine. Dr. Bruce Alberts and Dr. William A. Wulf are chairman and vice chairman, respectively, of the National Research Council.

Preface

In response to a request from the National Library of Medicine (NLM), and with support from the Warren Grant Magnuson Clinical Center of the National Institutes of Health and from the Massachusetts Health Data Consortium, the Computer Science and Telecommunications Board (CSTB) initiated a study in October 1995 on maintaining privacy and security in health care applications of the national information infrastructure (NII). As one of the lead agencies within the executive branch for facilitating the development and expansion of health care applications of the NII, NLM identified privacy and security as primary issues that need to be addressed in order to facilitate greater use of information technology within the health care sector.[1] Several reports written over the last two decades note the potential vulnerabilities of health information systems and the potential risks to patient privacy that could result from the

---

[1]The terms *privacy, confidentiality,* and *security* are used in many different ways to discuss the protection of personal health information. This report uses the term *privacy* to refer to an individual's desire to limit the disclosure of personal information. It uses the term *confidentiality* to refer to a condition in which information is shared or released in a controlled manner. Organizations develop confidentiality policies to codify their rules for controlling the release of personal information in an effort to protect patient privacy. *Security* consists of a number of measures that organizations implement to protect information and systems. It includes efforts not only to maintain the confidentiality of information, but also to ensure the integrity and availability of that information and the information systems used to access it.

unauthorized use of health data.[2] Although they outline risks and discuss possible corrective measures, these earlier reports do not attempt to evaluate the effectiveness of alternative mechanisms for protecting electronic health information. To remedy this situation, CSTB was asked to investigate the threats to electronic health information and to evaluate alternative technical and nontechnical means of protecting health information that are being used today. A natural outgrowth of this assessment is a judgment about the technical and nontechnical means that can be used to maintain privacy and security in health care information systems, about future research that is needed to develop additional mechanisms, and about the obstacles that stand in the way of future advances.

THE COMMITTEE AND ITS CHARGE

To conduct this study, CSTB formed a committee of 15 members and a special advisor with expertise in computer and information security, medical informatics, health information management, health care privacy, law, medical sociology, and health information systems. Both developers and users of health information systems were included. NLM charged the committee to do the following:

> Observe and assess existing technical and nontechnical mechanisms for protecting the privacy and maintaining the security of health care information systems, identify other mechanisms worthy of testing in a health care environment, and outline promising areas for further research.

In carrying out this charge, the committee was asked to address questions in the following areas:

> • *Threats to health care information:* What problems have health care organizations encountered to date regarding unauthorized access to individually identified patient data? To what extent has the security of health information systems been compromised or threatened by the introduction of electronic medical records and networked information systems? What problems could be encountered in the future related to unauthorized access to individually identifiable patient data? How sig-

---

[2]See National Institute of Standards and Technology, 1994, *Putting the Information Infrastructure to Work: Report of the Information Infrastructure Task Force Committee on Applications and Technology*, NIST Special Publication 857, U.S. Government Printing Office, Washington, D.C., May; Institute of Medicine, 1994, *Health Data in the Information Age: Use, Disclosure and Privacy*, Molla S. Donaldson and Kathleen N. Lohr (eds.), National Academy Press, Washington, D.C.; Office of Technology Assessment, 1993, *Protecting Privacy in Computerized Medical Information*, OTA-TCT-576, U.S. Government Printing Office, Washington, D.C., September; National Research Council, 1972, *Databanks in a Free Society: Computers, Record Keeping, and Privacy*, National Academy of Sciences, Washington, D.C.

nificant is the threat posed by inferential identification through the linking of databases with unidentifiable information?

• *Adequacy of existing privacy and security measures:* What types of policies are in place to provide privacy, security, and confidentiality? How adequate are these policies in practice? What technical features are incorporated into health information systems to provide security? How effective are they? What has been done to educate users about the need for privacy and security and their responsibilities for protecting health information?

• *Future mechanisms and best practices:* What other approaches to information privacy and security are worthy of testing in health care organizations? What approaches should be broadly promulgated? How cost-effective are various approaches? What combination of technologies, policies, and standards would help to promote better information security for health-related data? How can highly sensitive aspects of an individual's health care records (e.g., mental health history and HIV status) be better protected?

• *Barriers to adoption:* What barriers exist to the adoption of better information security practices and technology (e.g., cost, ease of use)? What incentives are needed to encourage providers to adopt sound information privacy and security practices and to secure health information systems?

Although the focus of the committee's charge was to evaluate practices that individual organizations can use to better protect electronic health information, the committee quickly learned from its research that the primary threats to patient privacy originate from the lack of controls over the legal (and generally legitimate) demands for data made by organizations not directly involved in the provision of care, such as managed care organizations, insurers, public health agencies, and self-insured employers. The committee regarded this larger threat as significant enough to warrant systematic attention. Given the committee's original charge and its composition, however, this report does not make specific recommendations in this area, although it does call for a national debate on these issues.[3] Accordingly, this report undertakes the tasks of raising consciousness in the health care industry (and the nation as a whole) regarding privacy and security issues in health care; demonstrating ways in which these issues can be addressed; and providing practical guidance to practitioners in the field of medical informatics and health information management who must continually wrestle with privacy and security concerns.

---

[3]Another study committee convened by the Institute of Medicine was charged to investigate systemic uses of health information and to offer recommendations in this area. See Institute of Medicine. 1994. *Health Data in the Information Age: Use, Disclosure, and Privacy,* National Academy Press, Washington, D.C.

Recognizing that organizations strive to balance security against other concerns such as cost and access to information, the committee investigated both the efficacy of various privacy and security measures and the implications of such measures for the ability of users to access critical information in a timely manner. In order that its work would have lasting value to the community, the committee attempted, where possible, to project future changes in the uses of health information, the potential threats to such information, and the technologies capable of addressing these threats.

METHODOLOGY

The committee's primary mechanism for gathering information about technical and nontechnical approaches to protecting electronic health information consisted of a series of site visits to six organizations that collect, process, and store electronic health information. Sites were selected on the basis of their reputed leadership in the development of electronic medical records, networked clinical systems, and privacy and security policies. Committee nominations were verified against reports or rankings in several highly regarded health care publications. The selected sites included a large, urban hospital; a tightly integrated health care system; a second tightly integrated health care system affiliated with a community health information network; a more loosely affiliated provider network; a state health care system; and a large insurer. To encourage personnel at the various sites to share their experiences candidly, the committee decided to keep sites' identities confidential.

Because site visits were conducted by different subsets of the committee's members, the committee as a whole developed a standard site visit protocol to ensure some degree of uniformity among the visits (see Appendix A). Prior to each visit, the site visit team gathered information from the site regarding its organizational structure, computer and data security policies, information systems, security mechanisms, confidentiality policies, procedures for releasing medical records, employee training and orientation materials, and disciplinary policies. This information proved valuable not only in orienting committee members to idiosyncrasies of each site, but also in indicating the degree to which the organizations had codified their policies and procedures.

During each one-and-a-half-day visit, the site visit team met with corporate executives; staff from the information systems, health information management (i.e., medical records), human resources, and legal departments; doctors; nurses; and other system users. Where possible, it met with members of health information management committees and of privacy and confidentiality committees. The site visit team discussed a wide range of topics with its hosts on each visit: confidentiality policies, policies regarding data exchanges and uses or releases of aggregated data, means of implementing policies, perceived and experienced threats to patient privacy and system security, training and education programs, information systems, electronic medical records, security mechanisms, users' perceptions of the information systems and security practices, and future needs.

In addition to its site visits, the full committee met five times during the course of the study to plan its work, listen to briefings from relevant stakeholders, and deliberate over its conclusions and recommendations. During these sessions, the committee met with health care providers, insurers, pharmaceutical benefits managers,[4] vendors of health information systems, experts in computer security (from both the health care and the non-health care communities), privacy advocates and consumer representatives, federal agencies interested in health information systems, insurers, relevant industry associations, and other organizations that maintain health-related databases. The committee also met with groups attempting to develop health care applications of the NII and with researchers who study the uses of medical information, including genetic information. Additional meetings were held with the Massachusetts Health Data Consortium and with representatives of European data commissions to understand the problems they face and the solutions they are implementing (see Appendix B for a complete list of people who briefed the committee).

The site visits and committee meetings provided committee members with numerous opportunities to observe and discuss the confidentiality and security policies, mechanisms, and practices used in a variety of health care organizations and firms in other industries. The visits themselves facilitated extended dialogue with key decision makers within the organizations, allowing the committee to better understand the objectives and motivations of the sites' privacy and security strategies. Many of the practices the committee observed during its site visits were described in its interim report released in September 1996.[5] This final report provides additional analysis of practices observed during the site visits and describes other practices that have not yet been applied in health care set-

---

[4]Pharmaceutical benefits managers are organizations such as Merck-Medco Managed Care Inc. and PCS Inc. that offer benefits plans that pay for prescriptions. They typically assist in designing the benefits programs, offer point-of-sale claims processing, and develop formularies of the drugs that participating pharmacies prescribe.

[5]Computer Science and Telecommunications Board, National Research Council. 1996. "Observed Practices for Improving the Security and Confidentiality of Electronic Health Information: Interim Report," National Academy Press, Washington, D.C., September.

tings; describes the general exchanges of health information throughout the industry and identifies obstacles to and incentives for increased attention to privacy and security concerns; and presents the committee's conclusions and recommendations on the state of practice today, on practices that should be more widely adopted throughout the industry, and on research needs for the future.

The committee recognizes that this report will serve multiple audiences: information systems and operations staffs within medical organizations who are charged with developing and implementing practices to improve privacy and security, government agencies and accrediting bodies with roles to play in overseeing health care organizations and other users of health information, and legislators and other policy makers who are interested in establishing a policy framework for protecing health information while allowing legitimate access. The commiteee hopes that each of these audiences will find useful guidance in this report, both in the detailed practices described in Chapters 4 and 5, and in the findings and recommendations contained in Chapter 6.

ACKNOWLEDGMENTS

The committee members that came together represented a number of different backgrounds and perspectives (Appendix E). The harmony with which people with such diverse points of view worked together is testament to the character of the individual committee members and a reflection upon the importance of the issue this report addresses. Each committee member volunteered a substantial amount of time over the course of the study to meet, conduct site visits, and draft sections of this report. To the extent that this report improves the privacy and security environment by enlightening the public, policy makers who set institutional priorities, daily users of health information, and those who build the systems, the committee members will believe that their effort was worthwhile.

To the CSTB staff, the committee expresses its admiration and gratitude for their faithful capture of the wide-ranging content of its deliberations and for the gentle but effective way they kept things on schedule. It is hard to find people of such talent who are willing to facilitate and support rather than impose their observations and conclusions. Thanks are also extended to those who volunteered to review and critique an early draft of this document, as well as to the numerous briefers who volunteered their time to meet with it and to help the committee better understand their concerns. The committee also owes many thanks to those who hosted the site visits. The committee received honest and open cooperation from a variety of individuals at each site.

Finally, the committee wishes to express appreciation to the sponsors of this report who were willing to invest in developing solutions to societal concerns: Dr. Donald Lindberg and Ms. Betsy Humphreys of the National Library of Medicine; Dr. John Gallin of the Warren Grant Magnuson Clinical Center; and Mr. Elliot Stone of the Massachusetts Health Data Consortium. Such leadership is crucial in motivating more than a fragmented approach to the search for solutions.

Contents

Whoever you are—
I have always depended on the kindness of strangers.

Blanche, in
A Streetcar Named Desire
Tennessee Williams

Executive Summary

Information technology promises many benefits to health care. By helping to make accurate information more readily available to providers, payers, researchers, administrators, and patients, advanced computing and communications technology can help improve the quality and lower the costs of health care. At the same time, the prospect of storing health information in electronic form raises concerns about patient privacy and data security, for although information technology allows the use of advanced technical mechanisms to limit access to health information, it also introduces new vulnerabilities.[1] Information technology facilitates both the storage of large amounts of electronic information in a small physical space and the dissemination of this information. It also enables the creation and analysis of large databases that contain information from various sources. Unless proper controls are in place, computer

---

[1] The terms *privacy, confidentiality,* and *security* are used in many different ways to discuss the protection of personal health information. This report uses the term *privacy* to refer to an individual's desire to limit the disclosure of personal information. It uses the term *confidentiality* to refer to a condition in which information is shared or released in a controlled manner. Organizations develop confidentiality policies to codify their rules for controlling the release of personal information in an effort to protect patient privacy. *Security* consists of a number of measures that organizations implement to protect information and systems. It includes efforts not only to maintain the confidentiality of information, but also to ensure the integrity and availability of that information and the information systems used to access it.

1

systems and networks can be accessed by unauthorized users. If not adequately addressed, such concerns can both dissuade health care organizations from investing in information technology and make patients reluctant to share information, undermining the provision of care.

In response to these concerns, the National Library of Medicine, together with the Warren Grant Magnuson Clinical Center of the National Institutes of Health and the Massachusetts Health Data Consortium, asked the Computer Science and Telecommunications Board of the National Research Council to examine ways of protecting electronic health information. As part of its research, the Committee on Maintaining Privacy and Security in Health Care Applications of the National Information Infrastructure assembled for this project conducted visits to six health care organizations that had demonstrated leadership in developing health care applications of information technology. This report examines the motivations behind the growing use of information technology within the health care industry; identifies related privacy and security concerns; and assesses a wide variety of mechanisms for protecting privacy and security in health care applications of information technology. As the report demonstrates, a variety of technical and nontechnical practices are available for protecting electronic health information held by individual organizations. Such practices do not address the privacy concerns that stem from the widespread and relatively unregulated dissemination of information among institutions in the health care industry, including providers, payers, researchers, and oversight agencies.

ELECTRONIC HEALTH INFORMATION:
USES AND CONCERNS

Information technology is becoming increasingly important to the health care industry as organizations attempt to find ways of lowering the costs of care while improving its quality. The health care industry spent an estimated $10 billion to $15 billion on information technology in 1996,[2] and further growth is expected as organizations implement electronic medical records, upgrade administrative and billing systems, install internal networks for sharing information among affiliated entities, and use public networks, such as the Internet, to distribute health-related information and provide access to clinical databases from remote locations. Much of the demand for information technology is driven by structural changes in the health care industry and its methods of care. Integrated

---

[2]Munro, Neil. 1996. "Infotech Reshapes Health Care Marketplace," Washington Technology, Aug. 8, p. 1.

delivery systems that combine hospital, clinic, and outpatient services in a single corporate entity share patient information between units to ensure continuity of care and reduce administrative overhead. Health maintenance organizations, which enrolled over 50 million members in 1995, demand information to analyze the outcomes and costs of different treatment plans.[3]

A central part of all these initiatives is the creation of electronic medical records (EMRs), which serve as the central clinical repository of information pertaining to patient care. In addition to streamlining administrative processes, EMRs hold great potential for improving care. Combined with analysis tools and decision aids, EMRs enable real-time review of diagnoses and care plans to ensure that established standards of care are being met. Properly implemented, this capability can reduce the variability in care and raise the quality of clinical decision making. The perceived benefits of EMRs among care providers have motivated growing investment in EMR systems—a trend that is expected to continue in the future.

Within individual organizations, electronic information systems and EMRs are potentially vulnerable to misuse from both authorized users and unauthorized outsiders who inappropriately access patient information for their personal or economic gain. Authorized users may take advantage of their legitimate authority to access information that they have no valid need to see (often regarding a friend, relative, or celebrity), or they may divulge patient information to others. Outside attackers may break into computerized information systems to steal, destroy, or tamper with data or to render the systems dysfunctional, preventing legitimate users such as doctors and nurses from accessing information critical to care. Health care organizations have experience in protecting against insider abuse because of their efforts to protect paper-based systems (though there is little data with which to determine the effectiveness of these protections). Provider organizations are considerably less experienced in protecting against outside attackers. As health care organizations expand the scale and scope of their computer networks, their vulnerability to outside attacks is bound to increase.

Little is known about the extent of privacy and security violations in health care organizations. During its site visits, the committee learned of only isolated instances of misuse of electronic health information, but no

---

[3]Pharmaceutical Research and Manufacturers Association. 1996. *Industry Profile*. Pharmaceutical Research and Manufacturers Association, Washington, D.C., Figure 5-3; available on-line at http://www.phrma.org. Also, Health Insurance Association of America. 1996. *Source Book of Health Insurance Data*. Health Insurance Association of America, Washington, D.C., Table 2.5a.

data exist with which to make more general assessments. Managers at most sites believe that EMRs enable them to control and monitor access to patient information better than they could with paper record systems. However, the expanding use of EMRs dictates that awareness of the privacy and security concerns must extend beyond the leading institutions the committee visited, to all potential users of EMRs.

Additional privacy concerns arise from the widespread dissemination of information throughout the health care system—often without explicit patient consent. Health care providers, payers (e.g., insurers), managers of pharmaceutical benefits programs, equipment suppliers, and oversight organizations collect large amounts of patient-identifiable health information for use in managing care, conducting quality and utilization reviews, processing claims, combating fraud, and analyzing markets for health products and services. In general, such information is collected for legitimate purposes, but few controls exist to ensure that it is not used for other purposes that may run counter to the patient's interests or patient privacy. For example, self-insured employers who collect patient data to monitor benefits programs and combat fraud are not systematically prevented from using such information to deny workers promotions or continued employment because of information in their health records. From the patient's perspective, the flows of health information among these many types of organizations may be of more concern than the possible misuse of information by authorized users within a particular organization or by outside attackers.

PROTECTING ELECTRONIC HEALTH INFORMATION

Protection of electronic health information held by individual organizations requires a combination of both technical and organizational practices, the selection of which involves implicit trade-offs among cost, complexity, and degree of privacy provided. Organizational practices are at least as important as technical practices. Although technical mechanisms can be used to validate the identity of computer users, establish controls on the information they can access, and encrypt information transmitted between locations, organizational policies establish the objectives of technical measures, determining who is allowed access to information and how tightly access will be controlled. Moreover, large numbers of health care workers have a legitimate need to access patient-identifiable information and have more opportunities than outsiders to disclose information inappropriately. As managers at several sites reported, strong training programs and disciplinary policies are often the most effective way of ensuring that workers comply with privacy and security policies. They act as a deterrent to potential abuse, rather than as an obstacle.

Such practices, however, do not address the privacy concerns stemming from the systemic flows of information throughout the health care industry. These concerns can be addressed only through initiatives at a national level that delineate and enforce standards for the appropriate uses of health information.[4] Existing federal laws, however, protect only data in the control of the federal government, and state laws provide inconsistent protection and often apply only to limited kinds of health information. In some instances, federal law facilitates the private-sector collection of patient-identifiable health information and allows self-insured employers to collect such information on their employees. Thus, to ensure the protection of health information, additional policy actions may be required.

As the site visits attested, health care organizations have a strong interest in maintaining privacy and security, but must balance this interest against the need to ensure that information can be retrieved easily when required for care. Many hospitals, for example, do not restrict physicians from being able to access records of patients not under their care, preferring instead to allow them access to information on all patients in case of emergencies. In some cases, practices have not been widely implemented that could improve security without adversely affecting care, such as systems for auditing access to clinical information or for systematically reviewing audit logs. Given the rapid pace at which health care organizations have been trying to install and expand the functionality of health care information systems, they have had limited resources to dedicate to security concerns.

Part of the problem is a lack of strong incentives for upgrading security practices. Privacy is not often a market differentiator in the health care industry; patients generally select care providers and health plans for reasons other than their ability to protect patient information. Because there has not yet been a widespread and public catastrophe regarding information security in the health care industry, many organizations believed that the risk of a major breach of security is low. Several sites visited for this study believe that they could survive a major event without significant consequences. Moreover, no strong legislation or enforceable industry standards yet exist that govern the privacy and security of health information. Thus, there have been few incentives to invest time

---

[4]These concerns are discussed in detail in Institute of Medicine, 1994, *Health Data in the Information Age: Use, Disclosure, and Confidentiality*, Molla S. Donaldson and Kathleen N. Lohr (eds.), National Academy Press, Washington, D.C.; and Office of Technology Assessment, 1993, *Protecting Privacy in Computerized Medical Information*, OTA-TCT-576, U.S. Government Printing Office, Washington, D.C., September, Chapter 4, pp. 75-87.

and money in efforts to significantly improve privacy and standards. Rising concerns about patient privacy—and recent legislative initiatives— may create new incentives for improving privacy and security within the health care industry. The Health Insurance Portability and Accountability Act of 1996, for example, directs the Secretary of Health and Human Services to develop and promulgate security standards for electronic health information by February 1998 and to make recommendations to Congress regarding the privacy of individually identifiable health information by August 1997. Other legislation was introduced to the 105th Congress that also addresses the privacy of health information.[5]

RECOMMENDATIONS

In order to better protect electronic health information, health care organizations will have to work individually, collectively, and with relevant government entities to address the broad scope of concerns regarding privacy and security. Choices will need to be made regarding practices that adequately balance privacy concerns against the need to ensure access to the information for providing care. The recommendations provided below reflect the committee's deliberations regarding feasible practices for improving the privacy and security of electronic health information at the level of both individual organizations and the health care system as a whole. They address several areas: privacy and security practices health care organizations should adopt to protect electronic health information; mechanisms for creating an industry-wide infrastructure for improving privacy and security; ways of addressing privacy concerns that arise from the systemic sharing of information among different institutions; development of patient identifiers; and topics for future research.

Improving Privacy and Security Practices

Health care organizations can adopt a number of technical and organizational practices to improve the protection of health information. Different health organizations face different threats and differ in the resources

---

[5]The Fair Health Information Practices Act of 1997 was introduced in the 105th Congress on January 7, 1997. During the 104th Congress, no fewer than three bills were introduced into Congress related to the privacy and security of health information, some of which may be reintroduced in the 105th Congress: S. 1360 (the Medical Records Confidentiality Act of 1995), H.R. 435 (the Fair Health Information Practices Act of 1995), and H.R. 3103 (the Medical Privacy in the Age of New Technologies Act of 1996).

they can use to address security, and so it is not realistic to prescribe a detailed set of practices for industry-wide adoption; however, it is reasonable to provide practice guidelines that can be adapted to individual circumstances.

Recommendation 1: All organizations that handle patient-identifiable health care information—regardless of size—should adopt the set of technical and organizational policies, practices, and procedures described below to protect such information. The committee believes the technical and organizational policies, practices, and procedures listed in Box ES.1 can be implemented immediately without too much difficulty or expense. The list should be adopted in its entirety to ensure that measures are taken to protect against the variety of threats to electronic health information and to compensate for the multiple vulnerabilities of health information systems. Nevertheless, each organization—and each department within each organization—will need to determine how best to implement each practice to ensure that an appropriate balance is struck between access and privacy in each location.

The committee believes that adoption of these practices will help organizations meet the standards to be promulgated by the Secretary of Health and Human Services in connection with the Health Insurance Portability and Accountability Act—or can inform the development of such standards. Penalties established by the act for violations of privacy or security are likely to motivate organizations that collect, analyze, and store patient-identifiable health information to implement such practices. Further, the committee hopes that external auditing firms will incorporate an evaluation of privacy and security procedures into their annual audits of health care organizations.

Over time, the technical solutions available to health care organizations for protecting health information will evolve—as will the sophistication of the threat. Health care organizations will have to upgrade their security practices as new technology becomes available. Box ES.2 describes technical measures that health care organizations could reasonably adopt in the future. Their ability to implement the technical practices recommended will depend to a large extent on the general availability of the relevant technology. Some products will become available only if health care organizations demand them.

Creating an Industry-wide Security Infrastructure

While individual organizations can take many steps to improve the security of health information they hold, the committee's site visits and experience in other industries suggests that additional efforts must be taken to facilitate greater emphasis on security at the industry level.

BOX ES.1
Security Practices Recommended for Immediate Implementation

This box summarizes a discussion of practices recommended in Chapter 6 of this report. Readers should read Chapter 6 in full for the complete detail, argumentation, and support for these measures.

Technical Practices and Procedures

Individual authentication of users. To establish individual accountability, every individual in an organization should have a unique identifier (or log-on ID) for use in logging onto the organization's information systems. Strict procedures should be established for issuing and revoking identifiers. Where appropriate, computer workstations should be programmed to automatically log off if left idle for a specified period of time.

Access controls. Procedures should be in place for ensuring that users can access and retrieve only that information that they have a legitimate need to know.

Audit trails. Organizations should maintain in retrievable and usable form audit trails that log all accesses to clinical information. The logs should include the date and time of access, the information or record accessed, and the user ID under which access occurred. Organizations that provide health care to their own employees should enable employees to conduct audits of accesses to their own health records. Organizations should establish procedures for reviewing audit logs to detect inappropriate accesses.

Physical security and disaster recovery. Organizations should limit unauthorized physical access to computer systems, displays, networks, and medical records; they should plan for providing basic system functions and ensuring access to medical records in the event of an emergency (whether a natural disaster or a computer failure); they should store backup data in safe places or in encrypted form.

Protection of remote access points. Organizations with centralized Internet connections should install a firewall that provides strong, centralized security and allows outside access to only those systems critical to outside users. Organizations with multiple access points should consider other forms of protection to protect the host machines that allow external connections. Organizations should also require a secure authentication process for remote and mobile users such as those using home computers. Organizations that do not implement either of these approaches should allow remote access only over dedicated lines.

Protection of external electronic communications. Organizations should encrypt all patient-identifiable information before transmitting it over public networks, such as the Internet. Organizations that do not meet this requirement either should refrain from transmitting information electronically outside the organization or should do so only over secure dedicated lines. Policies should be in place to discourage the inclusion of patient identifiable information in unencrypted e-mail.

Software discipline. Organizations should exercise and enforce discipline over user software. At a minimum, they should install virus-checking programs on all servers and limit the ability of users to download or install their own software. These technical practices should be supplemented with organizational procedures and educational campaigns to provide further protection against malicious software and to raise users' awareness of the problem.

System assessment. Organizations should formally assess the security and vulnerabilities of their information systems on an ongoing basis. For example, they should run existing "hacker scripts" and password "crackers" against their systems monthly.

Organizational Practices

Security and confidentiality policies. Organizations should develop explicit and clear security and confidentiality policies that express their dedication to protecting health information. These policies should clearly state the types of information considered confidential, the people authorized to release the information, the procedures that must be followed in making a release, and the types of people who are authorized to receive information.

Security and confidentiality committees. Organizations should establish formal points of responsibility (standing committees for large organizations, a single person or a small committee for small organizations) to develop and revise policies and procedures for protecting patient privacy and for ensuring the security of information systems.

Information security officers. Organizations should identify an information security officer who is authorized to implement and monitor compliance with security policies and practices. The information security officer should maintain contact with relevant national information security organizations.

Education and training programs. Organizations should establish programs to ensure that all users of information systems receive some minimum level of training in relevant security practices and knowledge regarding existing confidentiality policies before being granted access to any information systems.

Sanctions. Organizations should develop a clear set of sanctions for violations of confidentiality and security policies that are applied uniformly and consistently to all violators, regardless of job title. Organizations should adopt a zero-tolerance policy to ensure that no violation goes unpunished.

Improved authorization forms. Health care organizations should develop authorization forms that will improve patients' understanding of health data flows and limit the time period for which authorizations are valid. The forms should list the types of organizations to which identifiable or unidentifiable information is commonly released.

Patient access to audit logs. Health care providers should give patients the right to request audits of all accesses to their electronic medical records and to review such logs.

BOX ES.2
Security Practices Recommended for Future Implementation

Strong authentication. Health care organizations should move toward implementing strong authentication practices that provide greater security than individual log-on IDs and passwords, such as single-session or encrypted authentication protocols and token-based authentication systems (described in Chapter 4).

Enterprise-wide authentication. Organizations should move toward enterprise-wide authentication systems in which users need to log on only once during each session and can access any of the systems, functions, or databases to which they have access privileges.

Access validation. Health care organizations should use software tools to help ensure that the information made available to users complies with their access privileges. Such tools, now under development, will scan the contents of a medical record to detect and mask particular units of information that a user is not authorized to see.

Expanded audit trails. All organizations that store, process, or collect health information should implement expanded audit trails. By 2001, all health care organizations should be able to maintain logs of all internal accesses to clinical information, especially if they begin to demand audit capabilities today. In the longer term, health care organizations should pursue the use of technologies and products that support interorganizational (i.e., global) audit trails that allow all patient-identifiable health information to be traced as it passes through the health care complex.

Electronic authentication of records. To ensure the integrity of data contained in electronic medical records, all health care organizations that use computer-based systems to handle critical records and functions (such as entering physicians' orders) should use technologies for electronic authentication that will be capable of identifying individuals who enter or alter information in the electronic record.

Mechanisms to promote sharing of information about the vulnerabilities of health information systems and about practices for addressing these vulnerabilities could lead to long-term improvements in privacy and security throughout the industry.

Recommendation 2: Government and the health care industry should take action to create the infrastructure necessary to support the privacy and security of electronic health information. The comprehensive protection of electronic health information requires an institutional infrastructure that will develop and promote compliance with industry-wide standards for privacy and security and facilitate greater sharing of security-related information among organizations that collect, process, and store health information. Although health care organizations have strong incentives to adopt information technology, they do not necessarily have adequate incentives to develop the infrastructure necessary to promote privacy and security without support from government.

Recommendation 2.1: The Secretary of Health and Human Services should establish a standing health information security standards subcommittee within the National Committee on Vital and Health Statistics to develop and update privacy and security standards for all users of health information. Membership should be drawn from existing organizations that represent the broad spectrum of users and subjects of health information. The subcommittee should be empowered to advise and offer recommendations to the Secretary of Health and Human Services regarding (1) uniform standards of privacy and security; (2) exchanges of health information between and among health-related organizations; (3) limits on the data collection activities of different types of health-related organizations (e.g., how much information the insurance industry needs for fraud detection, how long such information may be kept); and (4) acceptable and unacceptable uses of health information for different types of organizations.

Recommendation 2.2: Congress should provide initial funding for the establishment of an organization for the health care industry to promote greater sharing of information about security threats, incidents, and solutions throughout the industry. Many sites reported that their attempts to improve security are limited by a lack of good information about the types of threats the industry faces, the types of incidents that have occurred, and the kinds of practices that other organizations have successfully employed. Establishment of an organization to facilitate exchanges of such information would provide a vehicle for improving the security of electronic health information as health care organizations increase their reliance on information technology and would strengthen the knowledge base for making policy in this area. It could be modeled after the computer emergency response team established at Carnegie Mellon University for Internet security (the CERT Coordination Center) and be called Med-CERT.[6] To obtain the cooperation of health care organizations, Med-CERT would have to maintain the confidentiality of incident information shared with it.

---

[6]The CERT Coordination Center is the organization that grew from the computer emergency response team formed by the Defense Advanced Research Projects Agency (DARPA) in November 1988. Its charter is to work with the Internet community to facilitate incident prevention, incident response, and communication during system emergencies. It attempts to raise the Internet user community's awareness of computer security issues and conducts research targeted at improving the security of existing systems. CERT[sm] is a service mark of Carnegie Mellon University. (Information on CERT is available on-line at www.cert.org.)

Addressing Systemic Concerns Related to Privacy and Security

Recommendations 1 and 2 (with 2.1 and 2.2) address actions to protect the privacy and security of health information held by individual health care organizations; they do not address the privacy concerns that result from the legitimate and widespread *systemic* flows of information within the health care system. Although the committee was not constituted with the range of expertise needed to render recommendations about ways to balance patients' desire for privacy against the social benefits that accrue from better access to information for health care, research, and other purposes, it does call attention to the existence of this conflict and recommends a national debate to determine how and to what extent greater control needs to be taken over these flows of information in order to protect patient privacy.[7] Only when this national debate takes place can policy be formulated properly.

Recommendation 3: The federal government should work with industry to promote and encourage an informed public debate to determine an appropriate balance between the privacy concerns of patients and the information needs of various users of health information. The objective of this debate should be to develop a consensus about the ways in which privacy concerns can be balanced against the legitimate needs of other users for patient-identifiable health information. If the result of this debate is a decision that the privacy interests of consumers should weigh more heavily in this competition, several legislative options could strengthen the hands of consumers. These include (1) legislation to restrict access to patient-identifiable health information based on the intended use; (2) legislation to prohibit specific practices of concern to patients; (3) legislation to establish information rights for patients; and (4) legislation to enable a health privacy ombudsman (described below) to take legal action against those who violate privacy standards (these options are explained in greater detail in Box 6.2 of Chapter 6). To further this debate, the committee makes five subrecommendations.

Recommendation 3.1: Organizations that collect, analyze, or disseminate health information should adopt a set of fair information practices similar to those contained in the federal Privacy Act of 1974. These practices would define the obligations and responsibilities of organizations that collect, analyze, or store health information; give patients the

---

[7]A recent committee appointed by the Institute of Medicine was specifically charged to address these issues. See Institute of Medicine. 1994. *Health Data in the Information Age: Use, Disclosure, and Confidentiality*, Molla S. Donaldson and Kathleen N. Lohr (eds.). National Academy Press, Washington, D.C.

right to demand enforcement of these obligations and responsibilities; and require disclosure of data collection activities to make the sharing of health information more transparent to patients. Such disclosure would educate patients about the flows of health data and their rights in controlling those flows, thereby facilitating the discussion of privacy and security issues and the development of consensus. The committee believes that personal awareness of privacy rights and potential abuses is one of the best countervailing pressures against the economic incentives that drive organizations to share information. Moreover, public awareness and concern may be an essential prerequisite to the passage of necessary legislation of any strength.

Recommendation 3.2: The Department of Health and Human Services should work with state and local governments, health care researchers, and the health care industry to establish a program to promote consumer awareness of health privacy issues and the value of health information for patient care, administration, and research. It should also conduct studies that will develop a series of recommendations for improving the level of consumer awareness of health data flows. Patients appear to be less informed than care providers and other users of health information about the various ways in which health care information is used, the potential benefits of such uses, and the implications for patient privacy. Having a neutral party educate patients would be a first step toward elevating the level of debate.

Recommendation 3.3: Professional societies and industry groups[8] should continue and expand their leadership roles in educating members about privacy and security issues in their conference discussions and publications. These groups represent a wide variety of health care professionals who must address questions of access and privacy on a regular basis. They would make good platforms for educating many of these professionals about patient privacy and ongoing initiatives in government and industry.

Recommendation 3.4: The Department of Health and Human Services should conduct studies to determine the extent to which—and the conditions under which—users of health information need data containing patient identities. Patients, providers, and other users of health information continually question each other's needs for patient-identifiable data. Limiting the use of such data to those cases in which there is a

---

[8]These include, but are not limited to, the American Hospital Association, American Medical Informatics Association, American Health Information Management Association, College of Health Information Management Executives, Healthcare Information and Management Systems Society, Computer-based Patient Record Institute, and American Medical Association.

demonstrable need would be a first step toward promoting responsible use of patient information and reducing concerns about privacy. Given its role in recommending privacy standards and its position as a neutral arbiter, the Department of Health and Human Services seems the logical organization to sponsor such a study.

Recommendation 3.5: The Department of Health and Human Services should work with the U.S. Office of Consumer Affairs to determine appropriate ways to provide consumers with a visible, centralized point of contact regarding privacy issues (a privacy ombudsman). This effort would provide patients with a centralized source of information regarding patient privacy and provide a means to field complaints from patients about alleged breaches of privacy.

Developing Patient Identifiers

The current effort to develop standards for a universal health identifier as mandated by the Health Insurance Portability and Accountability Act has potential implications for patient privacy.[9] While use of a common identifier for indexing patient records has the potential of improving the quality and reducing the costs of health care by making a more complete patient record available to providers, of facilitating the creation of longitudinal patient records for health care researchers, and of simplifying the administration of health care benefits, it could also facilitate the assembly of information about patients without their consent (e.g., the linkage of medical records with financial and employment records).

Recommendation 4: Any effort to develop a universal patient identifier should weigh the presumed advantages of such an identifier against potential privacy concerns. Any method used to identify patients and to link patient records in a health care environment should be evaluated against the privacy criteria listed below.

1. The method should be accompanied by an explicit policy framework that defines the nature and character of linkages that violate patient privacy and specifies legal or other sanctions for creating such linkages. That framework should derive from the national debate advocated in Recommendation 3.

2. It should facilitate the identification of parties that link records so that those who make improper linkages can be held responsible for their creation.

---

[9]The Health Insurance Portability and Accountability Act directs the Secretary of Health and Human Services to promulgate standards for a universal health identifier that will be assigned to each individual (i.e., patient), employer, health plan, and health care provider for use in the health care system.

3.   It should be unidirectional to the degree that is technically feasible: it should facilitate the appropriate linking of health records given information about the patient or provided by the patient (such as the patient's identifier), but prevent a patient's identity from being easily deduced from a set of linked health records or from the identifier itself.

The first criterion requires that the nation decide which types of record linkages will be legal and illegal and establish a legal framework to codify and enforce those decisions. The second criterion helps to make such a policy framework enforceable, perhaps by making a visible and overt act necessary to link information. Thus, illegal or unauthorized attempts to link information from various sources can be detected and traced, and guilty parties penalized. The third criterion supports patient privacy by requiring that the patient provide some information (e.g., an identifier) that can be interpreted as patient authorization for a linkage to take place and by preventing inference of the patient's identity from the information contained in any collection of records.

The committee recognizes that practical application of these criteria (the second, in particular) will be difficult given the current state of technology. Nevertheless, these criteria are intended to ensure that privacy concerns are explicitly recognized in the debate over universal patient identifiers. In the end, other criteria will also have to be considered in deciding whether and how to develop a universal identifier—to ensure that it will allow access to patient records as needed for medical care, research, and billing; that it can be integrated easily into existing health information systems; and that some sort of system can be established for distributing and managing identifiers. Balancing these criteria against the privacy criteria recommended above may not be an easy task. For example, whereas the Social Security number (SSN) would facilitate access, would integrate well into existing systems, and has a system for assigning and managing numbers better than most alternatives, it is not clear that it can meet the privacy criteria without modification.[10] Although originally developed as an identifier for Social Security records, the SSN is now widely used for banking, employment, driving, and medical records, as well as for tax purposes, making it easier to compile a wide range of information about individuals. Making a recommendation for or against use of the SSN or any other proposal for a universal health identi-

---

[10]The SSN is currently the basis of the identifier used in the Medicare program (Medicare uses the SSN plus another alphanumeric character) as well as many other health organizations. Even where not used as the primary identifier, the SSN is often contained in the medical record. The Department of Veterans Affairs prohibits the use of the SSN as the primary identifier within its medical system, although it is only now moving away from an identifier based on the SSN.

fier goes beyond the committee's charge and expertise. The committee notes, however, that the use of *any* universal health identifier raises many of the same privacy issues raised by the SSN. The question the nation must therefore answer is whether there are ways of attaining the presumed benefits of a universal patient identifier without jeopardizing patient privacy.

Meeting Future Technological Needs

As the threats to electronic health information become more sophisticated and health care organizations take greater advantage of information technology, additional technologies for security will become necessary.

Recommendation 5: The federal government should take steps to improve information security technologies for health care applications. Such steps would involve three areas: (1) technologies relevant to computer security generally, (2) technologies specific to health care concerns, and (3) testbeds for a secure health care information system. In each area, the federal government will need to work with industry and universities to determine which roles it can most usefully play.

Recommendation 5.1: To facilitate the exchange of technical knowledge on information security and the transfer of information security technology, the Department of Health and Human Services should establish formal liaisons with relevant government and industry working groups. Many information security technologies of value to the health care community will be developed regardless of the specific needs or demands of the health care industry. To take advantage of such technologies, the health care community needs to become more closely connected with other industries on the leading edge of security and the information security community so that it is prepared to adopt relevant solutions developed for other industries.

Recommendation 5.2: The Department of Health and Human Services should support research in those areas listed below that are of particular importance to the health care industry, but that might not otherwise be pursued. These technologies offer greater immediate benefit to health care than to other industries for protecting privacy interests and require specific attention and funding by health-related government agencies and industry. These include the following:

• *Methods of identifying and linking patient records.* Research is needed to develop a scheme for linking patient records in a manner that satisfies the three criteria for privacy outlined in Recommendation 4, allowing patient records to be easily indexed and linked for purposes of care and other purposes and impeding inappropriate linkages. This research should also address the extent to which a universal identifier is needed to facilitate improved care and health-related research and to simplify administration of benefits.

• *Anonymous care and pseudonyms.* Today, patients who wish to remain anonymous for purposes of care run a serious risk that the medical history information needed to provide quality medical care will be unavailable. Some approaches to solving this problem show promise for reducing the need to link patient records through the use of patient-specific identification, thus potentially mitigating the need for assigning patients unique, universal identifiers.

• *Audit tools.* The generation of audit trails typically results in enormous amounts of data that must then be analyzed. Automated tools to analyze audit trail data would enable much more frequent examination of accesses and thus make audit trails a more effective deterrent.

• *Tools for rights enforcement and management.* The primary unsolved technical problem today relates to secondary recipients of information: today's access control tools can effectively limit the primary (first-person) access of any given individual to data stored on-line, but they are ineffective in controlling the subsequent distribution of data. More effective tools for control of secondary distribution of data, such as rights management technology, would go a long way toward enforcing restrictions imposed by primary data providers.

Recommendation 5.3: The Department of Health and Human Services should fund experimental testbeds that explore different approaches to access control that hold promise for being inexpensive and easy to incorporate into existing operations and that allow access during emergency circumstances. The trade-offs between access to health information and the potential benefits and harm resulting from greater access are not well understood. Research is needed to better explicate the costs and benefits of various levels and types of information protection so that decision makers have the information they need to make wise choices. Testbeds specifically for testing the efficacy of various security mechanisms should be developed on the scale necessary (single department within an organization, a single hospital, or a network of organizations) to mimic the types of behaviors expected in an actual operational environment.

CONCLUSION

The committee believes that these recommendations provide a robust framework for addressing many of the vulnerabilities of health information systems at both the institutional and systemic levels. Clearly, additional work is needed, yet the committee believes that, with these mechanisms in place, the health care industry will be able to move forward in its attempts to improve health care while simultaneously protecting patient privacy.

1

Introduction

Protection of patient privacy is a long-standing issue in health care. Since the fourth century B.C., physicians have abided by the oath of Hippocrates, binding them to keep secret the information they learn from patients during the course of providing care.[1] Over the centuries, changes in the practice of medicine and in the structure of the health care industry have required a continuing expansion of the notion of patient privacy beyond the traditional patient-provider relationship and into other organizations that collect and analyze health information. Insurers, managed care organizations, public health officials, researchers, and others with a need for patient information have had to develop policies and practices for protecting the information they collect and, ultimately, the privacy of the individuals to whom the information pertains.

The growing use of information technology within the health care sector demands that issues of patient privacy and data security again be analyzed to ensure that policies, practices, and procedures for handling health information take into account the vulnerabilities these systems

---

[1] The pertinent part of the oath can be translated as follows: "Whatsoever things I see or hear concerning the life of men, in my attendance on the sick or even apart therefrom, which ought not to be noised abroad, I will keep silence thereon, counting such things to be as sacred as secrets." (Bulger, R.J. 1987. "The Search for a New Ideal," pp. 9-21 in *In Search of the Modern Hippocrates*, R.J. Bulger (ed.). University of Iowa Press, Iowa City, Iowa.)

entail.[2]   As health care organizations collect, process, and store more health information in computerized form and use both private and public telecommunications systems to transmit this information between different entities, they must ensure that adequate mechanisms are in place to protect the information.

This report investigates ways of protecting health information in an era of increasing computerization and far-reaching communications. It concentrates primarily on protecting patient-identifiable health information, that is, health records that contain information from which the patient's identity can be deduced or inferred.[3]   It assesses technical and organizational practices currently in use for protecting electronic health information, identifies other technologies worthy of testing in health care settings, and outlines areas for future research.   In addition, the report discusses the privacy concerns that stem from the increasing exchanges of information among different types of organizations involved in providing care, paying for care, or conducting analyses of health information for a wide range of societal purposes.   As the report notes, such sharing of information may pose greater privacy concerns than unauthorized access to health information stored at any individual location.

THE GROWING USE OF INFORMATION TECHNOLOGY IN HEALTH CARE

Expenditures on information technology for health care are growing rapidly. The health care industry spends approximately $10 billion to $15 billion a year on information technology, and expenditures are expected to grow by 15 to 20 percent a year for the next several years.[4] Health care organizations are developing electronic medical records (EMRs) for stor-

---

[2] The terms *privacy, confidentiality,* and *security* are used in many different ways to discuss the protection of personal health information. This report uses the term *privacy* to refer to an individual's desire to limit the disclosure of personal information. It uses the term *confidentiality* to refer to a condition in which information is shared or released in a controlled manner. Organizations develop confidentiality policies to codify their rules for controlling the release of personal information in an effort to protect patient privacy. *Security* consists of a number of measures that organizations implement to protect information and systems. It includes efforts not only to maintain the confidentiality of information, but also to ensure the integrity and availability of that information and the information systems used to access it.

[3] The protection of genomic data and tissue samples, while also of increasing concern, is not specifically addressed in this report, although much of the discussion of patient-identifiable information does apply.

[4] Munro, Neil. 1996. "Infotech Reshapes Health Care Marketplace," *Washington Technology,* Aug. 8, p. 1.

ing clinical information, upgrading administrative and billing systems to reduce errors and lower administrative costs, and installing internal networks for sharing information among affiliated entities. Organizations are also beginning to experiment with the use of public networks, such as the Internet, to allow employees and physicians to access clinical information from off-site locations and to enable organizations to share information for purposes of care, reimbursement, benefits management, and research.[5] Others are using the Internet to disseminate information about health plans and research.[6] The National Library of Medicine recently awarded 19 contracts to a variety of health care organizations across the country to investigate innovative uses of the national information infrastructure for health care, including telemedicine and information sharing (see Appendix C). Much of the demand for information technology is driven by changes in the underlying structure of the health care industry itself and its methods of care, as well as by concerns over rising health care costs. A central part of all these initiatives is the creation of EMRs, which serve as the central clinical repository of information pertaining to patient care.[7]

Changes in the Health Care Delivery System

The application of new technology to health care both drives and is driven by a fundamental restructuring of the U.S. health care delivery system. In recent years, the health care industry has seen (1) significant consolidation of providers and mergers of care-financing and provider organizations, (2) use of increasingly sophisticated management approaches to share financial risks for care between industry segments, and (3) new entrants into the market for analysis of clinical practice. This transformation is largely the result of pressures to reduce the cost of care, enhance the ability to measure and improve the quality of care, and move care delivery to less expensive settings. Overall, these changes have led to a significant increase in the collection and use of patient health data and in the sharing of these data across organizational boundaries. The

---

[5] *Health Data Network News*. 1996. "Claims Over the Internet? It's Happening," May 20, p. 1. See also Fisher, Lawrence M. 1996. "Netscape's Founder Begins a New Venture," *New York Times*, June 18.

[6] Fisher, Lawrence M. 1996. "Health On-Line: A Participatory Brand of Medicine," *New York Times*, June 24.

[7] Many terms are used to describe the electronic storage of patient-specific information; apart from *electronic medical record* (EMR), the two most commonly used terms are *computer-based patient record* and *electronic health record*. The committee chose to use EMR without intending to resolve the debates that surround the use of each term.

rise of health maintenance organizations (HMOs), for example, has increased demand for information about the outcomes and costs of different treatment plans. Continuation of the transformation over the next decade will force additional changes in organizations involved in providing and monitoring health care and in their demand for additional health information.

Integrated Delivery Systems

Integrated delivery systems (IDSs) are rapidly becoming the primary means of delivering care in the United States. Though their forms vary and will continue to evolve, IDSs generally consolidate under one corporate umbrella multiple types of care providers that serve different aspects of the care continuum (such as hospitals and primary care clinics). Some IDSs also include a health care financing arm that offers health plans and pays for care. A 1996 survey by Deloitte and Touche indicates that 24 percent of U.S. hospitals already belong to an IDS, and an additional 47 percent are participating in the development of an IDS.[8]

The move toward integrated delivery systems is motivated by promises of cost savings through consolidations, expansions of market share to protect current business, improvements in the quality of care by managing care over a continuum of time and encounters, and improvements in bargaining position with respect to payers. IDSs view integrated information systems as critical to achieving their objectives. In the Deloitte and Touche survey, 67 percent of the hospitals state that they are pursuing the development of an integrated information network. They anticipate that their capital investment in information systems will increase 27 percent over the next two years.[9] The investments will lead to a significant increase in the use of information technology to store, analyze, and improve access to patient health data. Access to these data is likely to expand well beyond the organizational setting that initially gathered the data to include sharing of data among providers and organizations that are members of the IDS.

Managed Care

Managed care programs, such as HMOs, are growing rapidly in the United States. In contrast to traditional forms of insurance in which care providers or patients are reimbursed for services rendered, managed care

---

[8] Deloitte and Touche LLP. 1996. *U.S. Hospitals and the Future of Health Care.* Deloitte and Touche, Philadelphia.

[9] Traditionally this investment in hospitals has increased 4 to 6 percent per annum.

programs use a capitation system to pay for health care and manage risk.[10] In a capitation system, providers are reimbursed based on the number of patients enrolled in their care (e.g., paid a monthly fee per enrollee) rather than on the amount and nature of services rendered. Between 1990 and 1995, total enrollment in HMOs grew from 36.5 million to 50.1 million, representing 20 percent of all private insurance.[11]

The rise of managed care programs has greatly altered the practice of medicine. HMOs have contributed to a shift in the view of medical care from mostly an art based on clinical judgment to mostly a science based on empirical data. Managing the practice of care now involves examination of aggregate data to define optimal approaches to the management of chronic diseases, for example, and analysis of the cost and quality of current and new care practices. Managed care providers emphasize the need to manage care across a continuum of encounters in addition to managing care within an encounter. As a result, managed care organizations have an opportunity to assess patient health risks and define optimal approaches to the management of the chronically ill, in addition to improving the efficacy of specific patient encounters with a health care provider. They also have an opportunity to use information about the health care needs of enrolled subpopulations of patients with common characteristics (whether gender, age, or condition) to improve care for individuals.

This shift has resulted in implementation of and experimentation with new data-intensive approaches to care provision and management. For example, the industry is developing measures of performance in the form of quality report cards administered by marketing or accrediting organizations. These include the Health Plan Employer Data and Information Set (HEDIS) developed by the National Committee for Quality Assurance and the Information Management standards established by the Joint Commission on Accreditation of Healthcare Organizations. In addition, providers are introducing more sophisticated approaches to managing the care of groups of patients with similar health problems (e.g., using demand management, disease management, and clinical pathways analyses). Managed care providers also tend to analyze the use of medical resources, including medications, specialists, radiology services, and sur-

---

[10] In practice, a provider may be wholly or partially capitated (e.g., it may be capitated only for the provision of primary care and paid on a fee-for-service basis for other care).

[11] Pharmaceutical Research and Manufacturers Association. 1996. *Industry Profile*. Pharmaceutical Research and Manufacturers Association, Washington, D.C., Figure 5-3; available on-line at http://www.phrma.org. Also, Health Insurance Association of America. 1996. *Source Book of Health Insurance Data*. Health Insurance Association of America, Washington, D.C., Table 2.5a.

gical procedures. Care providers and payers have begun to use total quality management and continuous quality improvement techniques to improve the quality of their services.

New Users of Health Information

Further fueling demand for information technology in health care is the entrance of new types of organizations that collect health information. These organizations typically provide products and services to the health care industry and have developed significant business interests that involve the collection of patient-identifiable health data. Examples include medical and surgical suppliers, pharmaceutical companies, reference laboratories, and companies that provide information technology services. Some of these companies have seen profit margins decline in their core businesses and see synergistic opportunities in the collection and analysis of patient-identifiable health data for health care organizations. For example, the pharmaceutical manufacturer, Merck and Company, acquired Medco, a pharmaceutical benefits management company that uses its database of medication claims to analyze utilization patterns for pharmaceutical products. Similarly Eli Lilly and Company, another pharmaceutical manufacturer, acquired the pharmaceutical benefits management firm PCS Health Systems Inc. Glaxo Wellcome Inc., a pharmaceutical company, has a significant interest in HealthPoint G.P., a developer of software for electronic medical records, to enable it to compare the effectiveness of its medications to that of others in treating various diseases and disorders. In many of these cases, specific agreements have been established to limit data sharing among affiliated companies, but the complex overlaps make security more difficult to ensure.

In addition, existing companies in the health care industry are expanding their roles. Several insurance companies have established their own provider networks. Aetna, for example, acquired a health care provider—U.S. Healthcare. Blue Cross and Blue Shield plans in several states are developing provider networks.[12] Providers are also moving into the administration and financing of care. One survey found that 15 percent of hospitals owned an HMO in 1996, compared to 10 percent in 1994.[13]

---

[12]See Auerbach, Stuart. 1997. "Two Blue Cross Plans in Area Agree to Merge," *Washington Post*, January 15, pp. C10 and C12. See also, Freudenheim, Milt. 1996. "Blue Cross Groups Seek Profit, and States Ask Share of Riches," *New York Times*, March 25, p. A1.

[13]Deloitte and Touche LLP. 1996. *U.S. Hospitals and the Future of Health Care.* Deloitte and Touche, Philadelphia.

The Electronic Medical Record

Central to the efforts of health care providers to integrate functions and shift to managed care is the development of EMRs. Fifty-six percent of hospitals were investing in EMRs in 1995; largely as a result of investments by IDSs, the market for EMRs systems is expected to grow 70 percent annually from $100 million in 1995 to $1.5 billion in 2000.[14] Virtually all of the sites visited by the committee in the course of this study were in the midst of developing an EMR system. The rapid movement toward EMRs results not just from changes in the structure of the health care industry, but also from general advances in information technology. The greater speed and power of information technology accentuate the advantages of EMRs over paper records, and the more widespread use of computers throughout industry has created an infrastructure for supporting their implementation.

Content of Electronic Medical Records

At present, EMRs represent an attempt to translate information from paper records into a computerized format. Over time, it is anticipated that the content of EMRs will expand beyond that of paper records and potentially include on-line imagery (e.g., x-rays) and video (e.g., a telemedicine session). For the time being, EMRs document patients' histories, family histories, risk factors, findings from physical examinations, vital signs, test results, known allergies, immunizations, health problems, therapeutic procedures and medications, and responses to therapy. They also include the provider's assessment and plans, advance directives, information on the patient's assent to and understanding of therapy, and permission for disclosure of information for use by other care providers or bill payers.

Originally, the medical record existed in abbreviated form to refresh the memory of the family doctor, who may have known more than patients themselves about familial risk factors and a patient's history of diseases or conditions. But because care is now provided by a variety of providers from a variety of locations and the bills are paid by more than one payer, the EMR is used to facilitate familiarity with the patient's status, document care, plan for discharge, document the need for care, assess the quality of care, determine reimbursement rates, justify reimbursement claims, pursue clinical or epidemiological research, and measure outcomes of the care process.

---

[14]*Health Management Technology.* 1995. "I/T Sales to Soar Next Five Years," December, p. 10.

Advantages of Electronic Medical Records

EMRs offer many potential advantages over traditional paper-based records. The primary benefit of using electronic records is access for authorized and authenticated users. EMRs allow providers to access health information from a variety of locations and to share that information more easily with other potential users. Multiple users may access the information simultaneously. When used to increase communication among providers, EMRs can reduce the number of redundant queries and diagnostic tests and improve the availability of health-related information at the point of care delivery. EMRs also offer opportunities for improving security. With EMRs, access can be limited to just that portion of the record that is pertinent for the user. For example, a radiology file clerk might have access only to radiology reports of all patients, whereas a physician might be granted access to the entire record of his or her patients. In addition, EMRs can allow all instances of access to be recorded in audit logs so that there is a record of who saw what information at what time and date on which patients.

To many organizations, increased access, better logical organization, and greater legibility are reason enough to justify the move toward EMRs. However, electronic data can also be used to accomplish tasks that are not possible in the paper format even if access were not a problem. For example, data stored in electronic records can be organized and displayed in a variety of different ways that are tailored to particular clinical needs. Electronic health information can be manipulated by computer-based tools, so that knowledge about standards of care can be used to generate alerts, warnings, and suggestions. These types of capabilities are known variously as real-time quality assurance, decision support systems, critiquing engines, and event monitors. Such capabilities may be useful in reducing some of the disparity between the amount and the quality of care delivered to different individuals. Electronic records also hold the promise of improving clinical research. Today most information about the effectiveness of tests or treatments, if in health records at all, lies buried in large stores of paper files that cannot be analyzed economically. The search and retrieval capabilities of computerized record systems, in conjunction with automated analysis tools, can enable much faster, more accurate analysis of data.

PROTECTING THE PRIVACY AND SECURITY OF HEALTH INFORMATION

The application of information technology to health care—especially the development of electronic medical records and the linking of clinical databases—has generated growing concern regarding the privacy and security of health information. Despite the enthusiastic reception of this enhanced capability for access by those who desire health information, many fear that transporting such information over the emerging national information infrastructure will further erode individual privacy. Coverage of health care privacy issues and public disclosures of sensitive data have become more common in the news media. Articles on the confidentiality of health information have appeared recently in the *New York Times*, the *Wall Street Journal*, and the *Boston Globe*. In a recent poll almost half of those questioned stated that they were "very concerned" about their personal privacy, and a third stated that they were very concerned about the possible negative consequences of EMRs.[15] Such concerns are growing as more sensitive information, such as HIV status, psychiatric records, and genetic information, is stored in medical records. Addressing these concerns requires both a better understanding of the vulnerabilities of health information in electronic form and the various mechanisms available for protecting such information.

Privacy and Security Concerns

The concerns of privacy advocates about electronic health information are based on two underlying notions. The first is that individuals have a fundamental right to control the dissemination and use of information about themselves. Because privacy is a fundamental right, advocates argue, other organizations that make claims on such information should be obliged to respect the wishes of the individual and to obtain explicit authorization from the individual for each instance of information collection, processing, or further disclosure.[16] The second concern is that information about an individual, revealed to some other party not willingly designated by the individual, may be used to harm his or her interests. These interests may include economic or social interests, and

---

[15] Louis Harris and Associates. 1995. *Equifax-Harris Mid-Decade Consumer Privacy Survey*, Study No. 953012. Louis Harris and Associates, New York.

[16] Note, however, that there are those who strongly believe that the decision to seek health care and to draw on medical expertise necessarily implies entering into a social contract to allow medical science and societal health to benefit from the use of data about *all* patients (provided suitable measures are in place to protect such data from inappropriate use). See Institute of Medicine. 1994. *Health Data in the Information Age: Use, Disclosure, and Confidentiality*, Molla S. Donaldson and Kathleen N. Lohr (eds.). National Academy Press, Washington, D.C.

they may or may not be tangible (e.g., disclosure may involve social embarrassment for which monetary compensation is not appropriate).[17]

Privacy advocates readily acknowledge that violations of a fundamental right to privacy or the uses of personal information that are harmful to an individual's interests do not depend on the existence of electronic health information—indeed, improper and harmful disclosures of personal information have mostly involved information taken from paper-based records. They argue, however, that electronic health information and computer networks compound the problem enormously.

Prior to the establishment of computer networks, health information had a physical embodiment, was awkward to copy, and was accessible only from central locations. The difficulty of moving health information increased dramatically with the volume of records being transferred. Automation and, more importantly, networking have changed this situation radically. Data have no physical embodiment, are easily copied, and are accessible from multiple points of access. Large numbers of records can be transferred as easily as a single one. The existence of the Internet means that data can be moved across administrative, legal, and national jurisdictions as easily as it can be moved to the next desk; intrusions can be mounted with equal facility. Electronic medical records also raise the possibility that much more accurate and complete composite pictures of individuals can be more easily drawn—so much more so that reasonable people would raise concerns about the aggregate even if they had no concerns about any single data element. Finally, any such aggregated database might well concentrate information in so lucrative a manner that the database itself becomes an interesting target for those seeking information.

Additional security concerns derive from the growing use of the World Wide Web. The spread of World Wide Web technology has precipitated a shift from a transaction-oriented approach to data transfer to an approach depending on a message-based client-server interface. In the transaction-oriented approach, users submit requests and receive responses in a stylized format. Because stylized requests and responses are limited in content to what style itself enables, not all data requests are possible, and expanding the scope of possible requests requires additional work on the part of the system developer. By contrast, Web-based interfaces are usually developed with tools that are intended to facilitate and improve system responsiveness to arbitrary user requests, and the

---

[17]Examples of information seekers include employers, government agencies, credit bureaus, insurers, educational institutions, the media, and private investigators. See Rothfeder, Jeffrey. 1992. *Privacy for Sale: How Computerization Has Made Everyone's Life an Open Secret.* Simon and Schuster, New York.

interface developer must work to reduce the scope of the requests that the user can make. Although a Web-based interface for examining data can be as restrictive as a system based on the transaction approach, checking whether a user's actions are appropriate is difficult and expensive; auditing a user's actions is more complex; and the assurance that the intended limits are indeed enforced is even more difficult to achieve. Nor is it necessarily possible to determine what the user intends to do with the information retrieved and if the user therefore is a threat to patient privacy.

The solutions advocated to address these privacy concerns fall into one of three categories. One approach is to forbid outright the collection of data that might be misused, on the theory that procedural solutions are inevitably ineffective and subject to abuse and compromise (these concerns about inevitable compromise are usually manifested in the area of secondary release of data). A second approach is to allow the collection of some amount of personal information (e.g., health information) under a specific set of circumstances but to impose on collecting organizations and parties rules about the management and disposition of that information and penalties for violations of those rules. A third approach is to specify conditions regarding the use of patient-identifiable health information through the policy process to which all handlers of that information are obligated to conform. The first proposal precludes the development of electronic databases of health information. The second two approaches can be implemented through the promulgation of appropriate public and organizational policy and the use of certain technologies. The second approach leads to situations in which the same information is handled differently by different organizations, simply because they fall into different categories. The third approach leads to a more uniform treatment of data and represents a high-level organizing principle for governing the protection of patient-specific information.

Addressing Privacy and Security Concerns

Even before the advent of computers, significant resources were devoted to the safeguarding of health information. Every accredited hospital in the United States had (and still has) a medical records department with responsibility for ensuring only legitimate access to health records, the integrity of data contained in those records, and the confidentiality of those records. Health care organizations established policies regarding the collection, use, and release of health information to maintain privacy and security, and they evaluated the relative costs and benefits of alternative mechanisms for protecting health information.

With electronic health information, the same issues still apply, though the mechanisms used to provide protection may be different. Health care organizations must decide who can have access to health information systems and whose needs for access are legitimate. Individuals assume that they have the right to keep information about their health private, yet most would acknowledge that health care providers need access to pertinent facts about a patient's history, test results, allergies, symptoms, and response to therapy in order to provide advice and make decisions that will be in the best interests of the individual's health. Others, such as researchers, health insurers, life insurance companies, employers, and marketers of health products, all have a legitimate need to access some types of health care information. Clinical researchers and epidemiologists need health information to answer questions about the effectiveness of specific therapies, patterns of health risks, behavioral risks, environmental hazards, or genetic predisposition for a disease or condition (e.g., birth defects). Health insurers seek to combat rising costs of care by using large amounts of patient data in order to judge the appropriateness of medical procedures.[18] Life insurance companies created the Medical Information Bureau Inc. to improve the underwriting process and help detect possible instances of fraud in the use of health information (Box 1.1). Drug companies want to know who is taking which drug so that they can conduct postmarketing surveillance to develop marketing strategies. A growing number of companies serve as information clearinghouses, collecting data from any number of sources and reselling it to customers in search of efficiency and savings.

In certain instances the desire for access transcends health care decisions and economic incentives. Foreign governments, voters, and business leaders are interested in the health of politicians, celebrities, and prominent citizens. A recent book, *Hidden Illness in the White House*,[19] and a recent film, *The Madness of King George*, are illustrations of the tension between an individual's desire for privacy and another group's claims of legitimate access to information concerning the health of its leaders. In Russia, one of Boris Yeltsin's surgeons acknowledged that Yeltsin had

---

[18]A recent news article described the payer point of view. "They [the privacy advocates and patients] think that we are seeking personal detail. But we're seeking clinical accountability. Ten years ago, there was no accountability. They sent in a claim and it was paid. Today, we ask for information . . . . " (Ian Schaffer, Medical Director, Value Behavioral Health, as quoted in Riley, John, 1996, "When You Can't Keep a Secret," *NY Newsday*, April 1, p. A36. The same article (at p. A37) describes a case in which a U.S. Circuit court of appeals concluded, "We hold that a self-insured employer's need for access to employee prescription records under its health plan outweighs an employee's interest in keeping his prescription drug purchases confidential.")

[19]Crispell, Kenneth A., and Carlos F. Gomez. 1988. *Hidden Illness in the White House.* Duke University Press, Durham, N.C.

failed to disclose details about his health status during an election campaign because his advisors felt that such disclosure would adversely affect the outcome of the election.[20]

Policies must be established to determine who can have access to what information. Organizations must then implement mechanisms to prevent those without legitimate needs from gaining access to information and must try to develop mechanisms to keep those who are granted access from divulging information to others. These mechanisms must balance the need for information against privacy; they must protect information while ensuring that health care will not suffer because someone has been unable to gain access to important information. They must reduce to an acceptable level the risk that health information might be used for purposes that harm (in a physical, emotional, or economic way) the patient, those who care for the patient, or the family and associates of the patient, while still providing legitimate access to ensure that the patient's care will not be compromised, payers will not be defrauded, and researchers can obtain information that will enable further knowledge. Finding the appropriate set of mechanisms for deployment within health care organizations is complicated by the fact that all access controls cost money and time. Care providers who have legitimate needs to access patient information must pass through access controls many times in the course of a day. If authentication and access pathways for users are inconvenient or time consuming, providers will generally choose convenience and may attempt to find ways to bypass controls or refuse to use a system with these pathways.

A variety of mechanisms exist for protecting electronic health information.[21] These include both technical measures for improving computer and network security as well as organizational measures for ensuring that workers understand their responsibility to protect information and for detecting and reporting violations. Understanding the efficacy, costs, and trade-offs between protection and access inherent in each of these mechanisms is central to implementing sound programs for improving privacy and security in the health care industry. By clearly delineating the types of privacy and security concerns associated with health information, reviewing the uses to which health information is put, and evaluating technical and organizational mechanisms for protecting health

---

[20] *CNN Interactive*. 1996. "Yeltsin Had Heart Attack During Russian Elections," September 21; available on-line at www.cnn.com.

[21] A bibliography compiled by the National Library of Medicine identifies some 800 recent references on topics related to the security and confidentiality of health information. See National Library of Medicine. 1996. *Current Bibliographies in Medicine: Confidentiality of Electronic Health Data*, No. 95-10. National Library of Medicine, Rockville, Md.

BOX 1.1
The Medical Information Bureau Inc.

The Medical Information Bureau (MIB) Inc. is a nonprofit trade association designed to alert member insurance companies of possible fraud or omissions in life insurance applications. The organization was founded in 1902 by the medical directors of 15 life insurance companies who were concerned that their companies had lost substantial amounts of money because of undetected fraud and omission. Today, MIB has 680 member life insurance companies, including almost every major issuer of individual life, health, and disability insurance in the United States and Canada.

MIB collects information about individuals from its member insurance companies. Member companies are required to submit reports to MIB regarding particular applicants if, in the underwriter's judgment, the application contains information significant to life expectancy, such as high blood pressure. Medical conditions are reported by using one or more of about 210 codes. Conditions most commonly reported include height and weight, blood pressure, electrocardiogram readings, and x-rays if—and only if—these facts are commonly considered significant to health or longevity. Five additional codes record nonmedical information that may affect insurability, such as an adverse driving record or participation in hazardous activities. MIB receives about 3 million reports per year, representing roughly 10 to 15 percent of all applications. It keeps records in its files for 7 years and has a database containing reports on approximately 15 million individuals.

When a consumer applies to an MIB member company for individual life, health, or disability insurance, the company may ask MIB whether it has a record on the consumer. If there is a record, MIB sends it in coded form to authorized personnel at the requesting company. The company may use the MIB report to detect attempts by applicants to omit or misrepresent factual information; it may not use the report as the basis for denying an application. As a matter of sound underwriting, such decisions are based on independent investigations that document medical and nonmedical information about the consumer. As a matter of law, the National Association of Insurance Commissioners (NAIC) Insurance Information and Privacy Protection

---

information that have been demonstrated in health care settings, this report attempts to demonstrate ways in which privacy and security can be maintained in health care applications of the national information infrastructure. The content of this report is structured to provide illustrations of practical initiatives that can be pursued by health care organizations and to allow a more informed public debate over policy.

Model Act, which is law in at least 15 states, explicitly prohibits the use of MIB reports as a basis for decisions. The NAIC act and the federal Fair Credit Reporting Act both require that insurers explain the basis for adverse underwriting decisions.

MIB takes a number of precautions to protect personal privacy while providing insurers sufficient information upon which to base underwriting decisions. MIB reports do not include street addresses, telephone numbers, or Social Security numbers. Insurers are also required to provide applicants with a written notice informing them that they may make a "brief report" to MIB, identifying the uses to which MIB and its member companies may put the information, and outlining the applicant's right to demand disclosure of information held by MIB and to request that errant information be corrected. In 1995, about 163,400 people requested disclosures from MIB, resulting in corrections to 348 reports.

MIB uses a variety of mechanisms to provide security. First, the computer system is "exceptionally user unfriendly." Second, each member has a computer terminal dedicated exclusively to activities approved by MIB. Each terminal has a unique identifying code; all access to MIB is documented, and all requests and transmissions are verified. The system will disconnect from the terminal if the identification code is not recognized. It disconnects after receiving an inquiry that includes the correct code, then dials back the requester, using another code, to establish the connection for transmitting the requested information. According to MIB, all of its 200 staff members are educated regarding expectations of confidentiality, and are limited in their access to the MIB code book, computer room, and database. Member companies must make an annual pledge to protect confidentiality and must adhere to a number of specific confidentiality requirements. MIB audits its members regularly to ensure their compliance with these requirements.

SOURCE: Medical Information Bureau Inc. 1995. *Medical Information Bureau: A Consumer's Guide.* Medical Information Bureau Inc., Westwood, Mass., September. Additional information from Neil Day, president, and James Corbett, vice president, MIB Inc., briefing to the study committee, May 1, 1996.

GOALS AND LIMITATIONS OF THIS REPORT

Objectives

This report attempts to guide the debate over the privacy and security of electronic medical information by evaluating practices for better protecting health information. To this end, the report has the following objectives:

1. Illuminate the various flows that characterize the movement of patient-identifiable data over time.

2. Evaluate practical measures that can be (and are) used today to reduce the risk of improper disclosure of confidential health information while providing justified access to those interested in improving the quality and reducing the cost of health care.

3. Analyze the types of privacy and security concerns that must be addressed.

4. Examine obstacles and impediments to broader implementations of the measures that are described in this report.

5. Highlight areas that will require further work in order to protect electronic health information.

This report takes as its point of departure the committee's interim report,[22] which described practices the committee observed in operational health care settings. It expands on the interim report by assessing the utility of these practices in health care settings and by identifying other measures that could be adopted by the health care industry to strengthen its protection of health information. No single organization has implemented all the practices described in this report (or the interim report), but each measure is judged to be practical and economical based on experience to date. Additional mechanisms that are not yet feasible for application to health care are also identified as research needs.

What This Report Does Not Do

The original charge to the committee called for an assessment of mechanisms to protect the privacy and security of electronic health care information. Technical and organizational measures can help to protect health information within individual organization in which some consensus has been achieved regarding who may have access to particular sets of data. Once the data leave the umbrella of organizational control, however, and flow into databases of prescription records, insurance claims, or epidemiological studies, organizational protections become less effective, and national policy becomes relevant. National policy is much more difficult to forge because of the strongly conflicting goals of diverse constituencies. *This report does not address the proper policy balance between access and privacy across all organizations. It does not settle issues that involve making value judgments about benefits compared to risks.*

A second limitation of this report concerns the pace of change of

---

[22] Computer Science and Telecommunications Board, National Research Council. 1996. "Observed Practices for Improving the Security and Confidentiality of Electronic Health Information: Interim Report." National Academy Press, Washington, D.C., September.

technology. Whereas today's information infrastructure consists of Ethernet and the Internet, tomorrow's will consist of widespread high-speed networks and hand-held devices connected to the national information infrastructure through wireless communications protocols. Many of the technical recommendations contained in this report will become obsolete as the technical environment changes. This report cannot predict the advance of technology. Although the recommendations contained in Chapter 6 do identify a handful of technologies that will become available to health care organizations in the near future (three to five years), no attempt is made to extrapolate beyond that point. Health care organizations and policy makers at the local and national levels will have to remain cognizant of technological advances and facilitate their adoption.

Finally, this report is based largely on a review of practices used at a limited number of facilities, supplemented by reviews of existing literature. Despite its efforts to address many aspects of privacy and security, the committee cannot claim that this report is comprehensive. Many other health care organizations are likely to have developed innovative solutions for protecting electronic medical information that are not described in this report. To the extent that such solutions may be applicable to a large number of other organizations, the committee hopes that health care organizations will attempt to disseminate the results of their efforts among the rest of the community in order to ensure more widespread use of strong protections.

With these goals and limitations in mind, the committee hopes that this report will provide a better understanding of the issues and assist in reducing the harm that could be caused by inappropriate disclosure of health information.

ORGANIZATION OF THIS REPORT

The remainder of this report presents the results of the committee's work, including its findings and recommendations. Chapter 2 discusses the current legal and regulatory environment for protecting health information, noting its limitations and recent initiatives under way in government and industry. Chapter 3 discusses data flows within the health care industry and describes the general types of privacy and security concerns that must be addressed. These include both the vulnerability of data held by particular organizations and privacy issues resulting from the widespread dissemination of data throughout the health care industry. Chapters 4 and 5 examine technical and organizational approaches, respectively, for better protecting electronic health information. These chapters review and evaluate practices within the health care industry (many of which were observed during the committee's site visits) and practices in use by other industries. They include technologies currently in use in other sectors of the economy (such as banking and finance) as well as those still under development. Chapter 6 contains the committee's findings and its recommendations for increasing the privacy and security of electronic health information.

2

The Public Policy Context

The privacy and security of health information is influenced by many factors that operate at the public policy level. In the United States, protection of health information is generally divided between coverage for records systems operated by federal or state government agencies and record systems operated by the private sector.[1] At the federal level, data protection measures are found in constitutional law, the Privacy Act of 1974, and a few statutes that regulate narrow areas of data use. State health record laws generally define the types of information considered confidential and the circumstances under which health information can be shared without patient consent (Table 2.1). Records held by the private

---

[1]Other countries have different frameworks for protecting health information that reflect their different cultures, histories, and political structures. While perhaps providing additional models for consideration in attempts to devise policy for the United States, it is not clear that these structures could be easily adapted to the U.S. system of governance or culture. Hence, they are not reviewed in this report. For a review of privacy policy in the European Community, see Schwartz, Paul M., and Joel R. Reidenberg, 1996, *Data Privacy Law: A Study of United States Data Protection*, Michie Law Publishers, Charlottesville, Va.; Schwartz, Paul M., 1995, "European Data Protection Law and Restrictions on International Data Flows," *Iowa Law Review* 80(3): 471-496; and Schwartz, Paul M., 1995, "The Protection of Privacy in Health Care Reform," *Vanderbilt Law Review* 48(2):310. For a historical review of international perspectives on privacy and privacy policies, see Aries, Phillipe, and Georges Duby (eds.), 1987, *A History of Private Life*, Vols. 1-5, Belknap Press of Harvard University Press, Cambridge, Mass.

TABLE 2.1 Existing Federal and State Protections for Health Information

Mechanism	Purpose	Limitations
FEDERAL PROTECTIONS		
Privacy Act of 1974	Requires federal agencies to publicly disclose the existence of government record systems; allows individuals the right to access information about themselves and to copy, correct, or amend records kept by the government; limits the purposes for which the federal government can collect or disclose information without consent.	Applies only to record-keeping systems operated by federal agencies or their contractors.
Freedom of Information Act of 1966	Allows individuals open access to federal agency records, except for those with specific exemptions.	Does not specifically address disclosure of information held by federal agencies.
Americans with Disabilities Act	Prevents public and private organizations from discriminating against individuals because of a disability.	Applies only to those conditions specifically defined as disabilities, not to all health information.
United States Code, Sections 290dd-3 and 290ee-30	Establish special rules of confidentiality for records of patients who seek treatment for drug or alcohol abuse at federally funded facilities.	Limited in scope to information about drug and alcohol abuse; apply only to federally funded facilities.
Medicare Conditions of Participation	Requires hospitals to have a procedure for ensuring the confidentiality of patient records and allows information to be released only to authorized individuals.	Does not address security mechanisms or evaluate practices.
Constitutional law	Interpreted as protecting the privacy of information about individuals.	Lower courts have not strongly enforced this interpretation.

TABLE 2.1   Continued

Mechanism	Purpose	Limitations
STATE PROTECTIONS		
Statutes	Establish confidentiality of the doctor-patient relationship and common tort remedies for breaches of confidentiality.	Statutes do not exist in all states and are not uniform across states. Most do not address the flows of information to secondary users.
Constitutional law	Interpreted as limiting the collection and dissemination of health information.	Rights are not clearly delineated and vary from state to state; they are difficult to enforce.
Common law	Prevents public disclosure of private records, defamation.	Generally limited to only widespread disclosures of information to the public or to disclosures to parties without a legitimate interest (i.e., not employers who pay for insurance coverage).

sector are covered under a number of limited laws targeted at specific industries.

In general, government and industry-wide protections are limited in scope. Most health information in the United States is collected and processed by private organizations, which are unlikely to meet the applicable threshold tests for state action. Constitutional protections for informational privacy are subject to interpretation and have not been rigorously enforced. Similarly, the Privacy Act sets rules only for personal data controlled by federal agencies. Other federal statutes that regulate health data processing focus on even narrower sectors of information use. As a result, most health data are entirely outside the protections of either constitutional or federal law, although with the passage of the Health Insurance Portability and Accountability Act of 1996 (Public Law 104-191), the public policy context for protecting health information is changing.

FEDERAL AND STATE PROTECTIONS

Federal and state laws attempt to balance the public's right to access information gathered by the government against the individual's right to protect personal information from inappropriate disclosure. Maintaining this balance is becoming increasingly difficult as technology provides new and improved means to collect, manage, and distribute data and as groups of citizens have developed conflicting desires to protect special categories of data and acquire access to data and information. Yet, privacy and access are not mutually exclusive. Systems can be developed that provide suitable protections against unwarranted uses of health information while respecting the need for legitimate access.

Federal Statutes and Regulations

Federal statutes provide one framework for protecting health information. The primary vehicle for existing protections is the Privacy Act of 1974.[2] The Privacy Act was designed to provide private citizens some control over the information about them collected by the federal government. It protects individuals from nonconsensual government disclosure of personal information. The act prohibits federal agencies from disclosing information contained in record systems to any person or agency without prior written consent of the individual to whom the record pertains unless the disclosure or further use is consistent with the purpose for which the information was collected. The Privacy Act contains the following key provisions:

- Individuals are given the right to know that identifiable, personal information is available in a government record system and to know what that information is used for.
- Individuals have the right to access the information, have a copy made of all or any portion of it, and correct or amend the records.
- The information may not be used for any purpose beyond that for which it was collected.
- No information may be disclosed to any person or to another agency without the consent of the individual to whom the information pertains, except for certain routine uses and other specific uses described in the law.

Agencies are subject to civil suit for damages that occur as a result of willful or intentional action that violates any individual rights under the act.

Health care facilities operated by the federal government, such as those operated by the Indian Health Service, the Department of Veterans

---

[2]Public Law 93-579, 5 U.S.C. §552a.

Affairs, and the Department of Defense, are bound by the Privacy Act's requirements regarding access, use, and disclosure of health information. The Health Care Financing Administration (HCFA) is also covered by the Privacy Act's requirements for information collected on Medicare beneficiaries. Contractors who operate a record system on behalf of a government agency are also subject to the Privacy Act, and their employees are considred agency employees for purposes of applying criminal penalties.[3]

The Privacy Act also allows individuals to request that amendments be made to their records if they believe them to be inaccurate, irrelevant, untimely, or incomplete. If the agency refuses to amend the records as requested, individuals may request a review of the refusal and, if the amendment is still not allowed, may file a civil suit in federal district court. The act requires that agencies publish reports in the *Federal Register* when they create or change a system of records. The reports must describe the categories of records maintained, their routine uses, policies on storage and retrieval, and other procedures related to their use, disclosure, and amendment.

Additional privacy protections are contained in the Freedom of Information Act of 1966, which governs public access to all records maintained by the federal government. The act was created to improve public access to government information and promote openness in government. The Freedom of Information Act provides that any person has open access to federal agency records, except those records that are protected from disclosure by one of nine exemptions to the act. Medical files, the disclosure of which would constitute a clearly unwarranted invasion of personal privacy, are specifically exempted from the act.

Two federal statutes establish special rules to protect the records of patients who seek drug or alcohol abuse treatment at federally funded facilities.[4] These statutes apply to oral and written communication of information containing the identity, diagnosis, prognosis, or treatment of patients enrolled in programs for education, rehabilitation, research, training, or treatment. They provide a high level of protection and allow only limited exceptions for release of patient information, including disclosure with the written consent of the patient. Because they have the full force of federal law, these statutes supersede state laws on confidentiality.

The Medicare program has also served as a vehicle for expanding privacy protections. The *Medicare Conditions of Participation for Hospitals* requires that "the hospital have a procedure for ensuring the confidential-

---

[3]5 U.S.C. §552a(m).
[4]42 U.S.C. §§290dd-3 and 290ee-3 (1988).

ity of patient records. Information from or copies of records may be released only to authorized individuals, and the hospital must ensure that unauthorized individuals cannot gain access to or alter patient records. Original medical records must be released by the hospital only in accordance with Federal or state laws, court orders, or subpoenas."[5]

In addition to these acts and statutes, multiple federal agencies have laws that also provide specific policies the agency must follow regarding types of data collected, how the data can be used, and how access to the data is managed. The procedures of other agencies, however, do not have specific statutory-based policies and thus must rely on common law tradition and the application of ethical decision making in these agencies.

Limitations of Federal Protections

Federal protections for health information have several weaknesses. Both federal laws to protect alcohol and drug abuse information and the Privacy Act suffer from a limited scope of influence. Federal alcohol and drug abuse regulations apply only to federal or federally funded facilities that offer treatment for alcohol or drug abuse.[6] The Privacy Act, perhaps the most comprehensive of the federal protections, for example, applies only to information collected by government agencies. Federal agencies, primarily the Department of Defense and HCFA, do collect considerable amounts of personal health information, but the majority of health records in the United States are collected and maintained by nongovernment entities and fall outside the jurisdiction of the Privacy Act.

The Privacy Act suffers from additional weaknesses as well. Individuals who do not regularly review the *Federal Register* find the notification system unnecessarily burdensome and ineffective. The act also fails to provide a government oversight mechanism, instead placing the burden of monitoring privacy and redressing grievances on the individual. Other critics suggest that penalties prescribed in the Privacy Act are inadequate and that the act mandates no specific measures for protecting privacy (e.g., it does not define technical mechanisms that must be used to ensure compliance).[7]

Constitutional protections have also been weakened by a lack of enforcement. The Supreme Court's major modern discussion of an informa-

---

[5] *Medicare Conditions of Participation for Hospitals*, §482.24.

[6] 42 U.S.C. §§290dd-1. See *Whyte v. Connecticut Mutual Life Insurance Company*, 818 F.2d 1005, 1010 (1st Cir. 1987); *Heartview Foundation v. Glaser*, 361 N.W.2d 232,235 (N.D. 1985).

[7] Office of Technology Assessment. 1993. *Protecting Privacy in Computerized Medical Information*, OTA-TCT-576. U.S. Government Printing Office, Washington, D.C., September, pp. 78-79.

tional privacy right remains *Whalen v. Roe*.[8] In *Whalen*, the Court accepted that the right to privacy includes a generalized "right to be let alone," which includes "the individual interest in avoiding disclosure of personal matters." Despite finding a theoretical right to avoid disclosure of intimate personal matters, however, in *Whalen* the Court allowed New York State to keep a computerized list of prescription records for dangerous drugs and to require physicians to disclose the names of patients for whom they prescribed those drugs. The decision balanced the social interest in informational privacy against the state's "vital interest in controlling the distribution of dangerous drugs." Finding New York's program to be narrowly tailored and replete with security provisions designed to reduce the danger of unauthorized disclosure, the Supreme Court held that the constitutional balance tilted in favor of the statute. Despite upholding the mandatory compilation and disclosure of prescription data, the Court left the door open to future restrictions in light of technical change, noting that it was "not unaware of the threat to privacy implicit in the accumulation of vast amounts of personal information in computerized data banks or other massive government files." In so doing, the Court set the stage for claims that the Constitution embodies a right to informational privacy, although the Court has yet to expand on this idea in any significant way.[9] Despite the considerable power of the decision, lower courts have not capitalized on this constitutional doctrine's promise for improving health care privacy.[10]

Weaknesses also exist in the Americans with Disabilities Act (ADA).[11] This statute has proven less than efficacious in protecting medical privacy. To begin with, health information per se is not covered by this law. Rather, the ADA's applicability turns on whether or not an impairing condition fits among those conditions that have been found to fall within

---

[8] 429 U.S. 589 (1977).

[9] 429 U.S. 599-604 (1977). An alternative view is provided by A. Michael Froomkin (see "Flood Control on the Information Ocean: Living With Anonymity, Digital Cash, and Distributed Databases," available on the World Wide Web at www.law.miami.edu/~froomkin/articles/oceanno.htm).

[10] See, for example, *Doe v. Attorney General*, 941 F.2d 780, 795 (9th Cir. 1991); *American Civil Liberties Union v. Mississippi*, 911 F.2d 1066, 1069-1070 (5th Cir. 1990); *Walls v. City of Petersburg*, 895 F.2d 188, 192-194 (4th Cir. 1990); *Gitorerrez v. Lynch*, 826 F.2d 1534, 1539 (6th Cir. 1987); *Mann v. University of Cincinnati*, 824 F.Supp. 1190, 1198-1199 (S.D. Ohio 1993); *Doe v. Borough of Barrington*, 729 F.Supp. 376, 382 (D.N.J. 1990).

[11] 42 U.S.C. §§12111-12117. See Miller, Frances H., and Philip A. Huvos. 1994. "Genetic Blueprints, Employer Cost-Cutting, and the Americans with Disabilities Act," *Administrative Law Review* 46(369):383. ("Disabilities law has not yet caught up with the recent explosion in genetic technology that now facilitates testing for a wide range of genetic anomalies potentially detrimental to employee health.")

this statute's definition of "disability."[12]   Another limitation of the ADA concerns its lack of practical impact: job applicants and employees are often either unaware or unable to prove that employers have made decisions based on the health information about their employees.[13] The ADA may, however, sometimes provide privacy protection by making some employers reluctant to collect and process certain kinds of personal information. Because of fear of litigation, employers may avoid collection of data regarding health conditions that place an employee or a qualified job applicant under the ADA's protection. Collecting such data might lead to inference of an ADA violation.

State Statutes and Regulations

At the state level, measures for protecting health information include constitutional law and statutes. Constitutional law has sometimes been interpreted as setting limits on the collection and dissemination of health data.[14] Statutory measures establish doctor-patient confidentiality and common law tort remedies.[15] More than a dozen states have enacted laws that place limitations on the use of genetic information by health insurers.[16]

States have specific laws that govern how open the records of the state will be, and many state agencies have agency-specific statutes governing confidentiality, access, and use of their data. However, little uniformity exists among state statutes and regulations protecting health information. Protections vary according to the holder of the information

---

[12]42 U.S.C. §12112(a). See Rothstein, Mark A. 1992. "Genetic Discrimination in Employment and the Americans with Disabilities Act," *Houston Law Review* 29(23):83. ("The ADA's coverage of a wide range of genetic conditions is not resolved.")

[13]See generally Burgdorf, Jr., Robert L. 1991. "The Americans with Disabilities Act," *Harvard C.R.-C.L. Law Review* 26(413):434-437. See also Schultz, Ellen E. 1994. "Open Secrets: Medical Data Gathered by Firms Can Prove Less Than Confidential," *Wall Street Journal*, May 18, p. A1.

[14]California Constitution, Art. I, §1. For cases interpreting this right, see *Urbaniak v. Newtown*, 226 Cal. App. 3d 1128, 277 Cal. Rptr. 354, 357-358 (1991); *Division of Medical Quality v. Gherardini*, 93 Cal. App. 669. 156 Cal. Rptr. 55, 61-62 (1979).

[15]See, for example, California Civil Code §56; Wisconsin Statutes Annotated §146.82; Rhode Island General Laws § 5-37-9. For cases interpreting the duty of confidentiality, see *Horne v. Patton*, 291 Ala. 701, 287 S.2d 824, 827-830 (1974); *Hague v. Williams*, 37 N.J. 328, 181 A.2d 345, 347-349 (1962). See also Gellman, Robert. 1984. "Prescribing Privacy: The Uncertain Role of the Physician in the Protection of Patient Privacy," *North Carolina Law Review* 62(255):274-278.

[16]For an overview and excellent analysis, see Rothenberg, Karen H., 1995, "Genetic Information and Health Insurance: State Legislative Approaches," *Journal of Law, Medicine, and Ethics* 23(312):312-319.

and the type of information (i.e., mental health, HIV or AIDS, substance abuse, genetic information). Most statutes do not address redisclosure of health information and lack penalties for misuse or misappropriation. Few states have enacted statutes and regulations as to whether medical records can be created, authenticated, and stored electronically. Only 28 states explicitly protect and ensure the rights of patients to review their medical records so that they can see what information exists about them and recommend changes or make amendments if necessary. Four states allow patient access to hospital records only, whereas 24 provide access to hospital and physician records.

As health care providers have expanded their reach across state borders, the need for greater uniformity has increased. In recent years, the National Conference of Commissioners on Uniform State Laws developed the Uniform Healthcare Information Act in an attempt to stimulate uniformity among states on health care information management issues. As of 1996, only two states, Montana and Washington, had enacted this model legislation.[17] Clearly, efforts must be directed toward developing national standards of confidentiality and security to support the development of computer-based patient record systems and to instill trust by consumers in the use of technology.

Limitations of State Protections

For the most part, state law has not overcome the weaknesses in current federal data protection. State statutes do not address the flow of health information to secondary users outside the provider setting. They do not address the responsibilities of third-party payers in handling health information, nor do they impose rules on the use of health information by secondary users of the data. Most state statutes fail to recognize the particular challenges posed by the use of electronic health records and by the rapid growth of organizations that compile information about patients—in both patient-identifiable and aggregated form—for sale to interested corporations.[18]

---

[17]The main provisions of this model legislation are (1) to give patients the right to have access to their own medical records; (2) to allow patients to correct or amend their records if the content is suspected to be in error; (3) to require providers to obtain a written authorization before disclosing patient information to other parties; and (4) to outline situations in which patient information may be disclosed without patient authorization. (gopher://leginfo.leg.wa.gov:70/00/pub/rcw/title_70).

[18]Office of Technology Assessment. 1993. *Protecting Privacy in Computerized Medical Information*, OTA-TCT-576. U.S. Government Printing Office, Washington, D.C., September, pp. 43-44.

The state legislative approaches to genetic privacy currently focus narrowly on genetic tests rather than genetic information that is generated in other ways.[19] In addition, the practice and administration of medicine now increasingly take place on an interstate level, which makes state solutions to data protection increasingly unwieldy.

The weaknesses of these state solutions become even clearer when one considers the common law right of privacy. One branch of this interest has been found to prevent public disclosure of private records.[20] Most courts have, however, found that such a claim requires widespread disclosure to the public, which will not occur in most cases involving the release of health information.[21] Another restrictive element of the public disclosure tort is that most courts define disclosure as the release of information to someone without a "legitimate interest" in the information. Some courts have found employers to have a legitimate interest in their employees' health information.[22]

A second branch of the tort right of privacy prevents intentional intrusions on the private affairs or concerns of an individual.[23] Such intrusion must be "highly offensive"; moreover, something in the nature of "prying or intrusion" must occur.[24] Courts have failed to find that disclosure of sensitive health information by an employer to an individual's coworkers creates such an intrusion; the employee had, after all, "voluntarily" provided the information to her employer.[25]

State protection of health information is further limited by the federal Employee Retirement and Income Security Act (ERISA). This law preempts state regulation of companies that provide health care benefits

---

[19]Rothenberg, Karen H. 1995. "Genetic Information and Health Insurance: State Legislative Approaches," *Journal of Law, Medicine, and Ethics* 23(312):312-319.

[20]American Law Institute. 1976. *Restatement (Second) of the Law of Torts*, §652D.

[21]*Porten v. University of San Francisco*, 64 Cal. App. 3d 825, 134 Cal. Rptr. 839, 841 (1976). For criticisms of the requirement of widespread publication, see *Miller v. Motorola*, 202 Ill. App. 3d 976, 560 N.E.2d 900, 902 (1990). See also Keeton, W. Page (ed.) 1984. *Prosser and Keeton on the Law of Torts*. West Publishing Company, St. Paul, Minn., §117 at 857-858.

[22]Keeton, W. Page (ed.) 1984. *Prosser and Keeton on the Law of Torts*. West Publishing Company, St. Paul, Minn., §117 at 857-858.

[23]American Law Institute. 1976. *Restatement (Second) of the Law of Torts*, §652B.

[24]Keeton, W. Page (ed.) 1984. *Prosser and Keeton on the Law of Torts*. West Publishing Company, St. Paul, Minn., §117 at 855.

[25]Miller v. Motorola, 202 Ill. App. 3d 976, 560 N.E.2d 900, 903 (1990). See Mares v. Conagra, 971 F.2d 492, 496-497 (10th Cir. 1992) (request of employer for worker to supply it with detailed medication information does not constitute a "substantial interference with her seclusion").

through self-insurance.[26] Due to weak federal protection, ERISA creates a considerable loophole for self-insured companies, which are not restricted from gaining access to personally identifiable health information pertaining to their employees. Over 60 million Americans held health insurance through a self-insured employer in 1993.[27]

NONGOVERNMENTAL INITIATIVES

Outside of government, a number of initiatives are under way to develop industry-wide standards for the security and confidentiality of health information. These efforts span a wide range of topics, from attempts to develop technical standards for security, to models for evaluating existing practices, to educational initiatives. They are being conducted by a large number of organizations, including the American National Standards Institute, the Computer-based Patient Record Institute, and the Joint Commission on Accreditation of Healthcare Organizations. While moving in the right direction, these efforts have not yet resulted in a set of enforceable standards that have been broadly adopted by industry.

American National Standards Institute

To facilitate the development of standards for health care information systems, the American National Standards Institute (ANSI) has established the Health Informatics Standards Board (HISB). Its charter is to promulgate standards for (1) health care models and electronic health records; (2) the interchange of health data, images, sounds, and signals within and among health care organizations; (3) health care codes and terminology; (4) communication with diagnostic instruments and health care devices; (5) representation and communication of health care protocols, knowledge, and statistical databases; (6) privacy, confidentiality, and security of medical information; and (7) other areas of concern or interest regarding health information.[28] HISB coordinates the work of standards groups for health care data interchange, such as the Institute of Electrical and Electronics Engineers, the American Society for Testing and Materi-

---

[26] ERISA, §502(a), codified at 29 U.S.C. §1132. See Bobinski, Mary Anne. 1990. "Unhealthy Federalism," U.C. Davis Law Review 24(255). See also Rothstein, Mark A. 1992. "Genetic Discrimination in Employment and the Americans with Disabilities Act," Houston Law Review 29(23):80-81.

[27]Health Insurance Association of America. 1996. *Source Book of Health Insurance Data.* Health Insurance Association of America, Washington, D.C., Table 2.5.

[28]American National Standards Institute (ANSI), Healthcare Informatics Standards Planning Panel. 1992. "Charter Statement," ANSI, September.

als, and the International Organization for Standardization (ISO). Its goal is to develop a unified set of standards that are compatible with the ISO and other bodies. HISB does not write standards or make technical determinations but instead coordinates the activities of other accredited standards bodies. Its voting membership consists of private companies, government agencies, individual experts, and other organizations. It includes users and producers of health information, professional and trade organizations, government agencies, and standards organizations.

Computer-based Patient Record Institute

The Computer-based Patient Record Institute (CPRI) is an organization of public and private entities that promotes the use of electronic health records. CPRI has recognized the importance of providing for information security in the implementation of computer-based patient records and has established the Work Group on Confidentiality, Privacy, and Security. The work group was chartered to encourage the creation of policies and mechanisms to protect patient and caregiver privacy and to ensure information security. As part of its efforts, the work group is developing a series of security guidelines for organizations implementing electronic medical record systems. Products issued to date include guidelines for (1) establishing information security policies, (2) establishing information security education programs, (3) managing information security programs, and (4) establishing confidentiality statements and agreements.[29] It has also developed a guide to security features for health information systems.[30] The thrust of these initiatives is purely educational. CPRI has no mechanism or authority to ensure compliance with the guidelines it promulgates.

Joint Commission on Accreditation of Healthcare Organizations

The Joint Commission on Accreditation of Healthcare Organizations (JCAHO) certifies the compliance of hospitals with a number of specific accreditation standards. The 1996 JCAHO *Accreditation Manual for Hospi-*

---

[29]Computer-based Patient Record Institute (CPRI). 1995. *Guidelines for Establishing Information Security Policies at Organizations Using Computer-based Patient Record Systems.* CPRI, Schaumburg, Ill., February. Also, Computer-based Patient Record Institute. 1995. Guidelines for Information Security Education Programs at Organizations Using Computer-based Patient Record Systems. CPRI, Schaumburg, Ill., June.

[30]Computer-based Patient Record Institute. 1996. *Security Features for Computer-based Patient Record Systems.* CPRI, Schaumburg, Ill, September.

tals specifies information management (IM) standards. IM.2 states that the "confidentiality, security and integrity of data and information are maintained." IM.2.2 states that "the hospital determines appropriate levels of security and confidentiality for data and information . . . " and continues by stating that the "collection, storage and retrieval systems are designed to allow timely and easy use of data and information without compromising its security and confidentiality." IM.2.2.3 states that "records and information are protected against loss, destruction, tampering and unauthorized access or use."

The intent of these standards is to ensure that a hospital maintains the security and confidentiality of data and is especially careful about preserving the confidentiality of sensitive data. The hospital is expected to determine the level of security and confidentiality maintained for different types of information. Access to each category of information is based on need and defined by job title and function.

According to the JCAHO, an effective process defines the following:

1. Who has access to information;
2. The information to which an individual has access;
3. The user's obligation to keep information confidential;
4. When release of health information or removal of the medical record is permitted;
5. How information is protected against unauthorized intrusion, corruption, or damage; and
6. The process followed when confidentiality and security are violated.

JCAHO examines hospital practices in the area of information management during its triennial reviews. The reviews address information management practices at an overall level but do not directly ascertain the occurrence of specific instances in which hospital practices may have been violated. JCAHO reviews are nominally voluntary, but organizations that participate in the Medicare and Medicaid programs (and expect to be reimbursed for services offered under these programs) are required to receive JCAHO accreditation.

IMPROVING PUBLIC POLICY

Better protection of electronic health information will require efforts at the national level. The lack of uniform national standards for the privacy and security of health information creates particular problems for health care organizations that serve constituents in multiple states and creates additional confusion for patients regarding their rights. The results are administrative uncertainty and potential violations of privacy in states with weaker confidentiality requirements. To further compound the problem, few mechanisms exist, inside or outside government, for monitoring and enforcing compliance with laws, regulations, and standards governing the confidentiality of health information. In particular, an individual whose information has been compromised generally lacks recourse for a specific incident and cannot receive compensation or ensure that those responsible for the incident are punished.

Conflicting views of data ownership and a lack of patient understanding of health data flows and of their rights to privacy and confidentiality also need to be addressed at a national rather than an institutional or organizational level. As site visits and briefings to the committee attest, patients, providers, health researchers, and other users of health information often have conflicting views regarding the ownership of identifiable health information. Patients tend to believe that information about their health history, diagnosis, and treatment belongs to them because it is about them. Health care organizations believe patient health information belongs to them because they invest resources in collecting, storing, and analyzing it and because they are required to collect data regarding patient care. Insurance companies, pharmaceutical manufacturers, and market research companies claim some ownership rights because of their vested interests. In addition, there is evidence that vendors of medical diagnostic equipment believe the data collected by their instruments belong to them because their devices have enabled its collection. The resulting confusion has frustrated efforts to enhance the privacy and security of health information by frustrating efforts to determine responsibility for protecting information.

Building National Consensus

Over the past several years, a consensus has emerged within Congress and among the general public regarding the need for federal legislation to address this important issue. The Office of Technology Assessment (OTA), in its report *Protecting Privacy in Computerized Medical Information*,[31] found that current laws, in general, do not provide consistent, comprehensive protection of health information confidentiality. Focusing on the impact of computer technology, the report concluded that computerization reduces some concerns about the privacy of health infor-

---

[31]Office of Technology Assessment. 1993. *Protecting Privacy in Computerized Medical Information*, OTA-TCT-576. U.S. Government Printing Office, Washington, D.C., September.

mation while increasing others. A 1994 Institute of Medicine report[32] recommends that federal preemptive legislation be enacted to establish uniform requirements for the preservation of confidentiality and the protection of privacy rights for health data about individuals. A more recent OTA report[33] identifies the issues of privacy and confidentiality as particularly important areas in dealing with health information. The report suggests that if there is little confidence that electronic medical information systems will protect them, providers and patients will be unwilling to use them. The report concludes that Congress may wish to establish federal legislation and regulation to protect medical information, as well as electronic data standards for storage and transmission of medical information.

As these reports recognize, legal regulation of medical privacy cannot focus solely on the doctor-patient relationship or the site at which the information is processed or stored. Moreover, an individual's own control over his or her health information cannot be complete because these data are essential for the modern distribution of health care services. In the computer age, health data pass through an increasing number of professional settings and organizations. The processing of personal information already plays a critical role in the provision, regulation, and financing of health services by government and private entities. Beyond the traditional doctor-patient relationship and the provision of health services in hospitals, a variety of public and private organizations now use personal health data. Moreover, health care reform will further increase the extent to which health care data are applied and shared. As part of this process, greater use will be made of information technology in an attempt to control costs and increase the quality of care.

In preparing and implementing laws and policies to provide privacy, policy makers cannot ignore the possibility that individuals may be discriminated against on the basis of specific illnesses or conditions they have or that sensitive or adverse information may be used against an individual's economic interests in some way. For example, an employer may refuse to hire or promote an individual with a long and expensive history of medical claims (or with the prospect of probable expensive or chronic medical problems in the future based on family history). Policy makers must assume that such discrimination is likely to continue in the

---

[32]Institute of Medicine. 1994. *Health Data in the Information Age: Use, Disclosure, and Privacy*, Molla S. Donaldson and Kathleen N. Lohr (eds.). National Academy Press, Washington, D.C.

[33]Office of Technology Assessment. 1995. *Bringing Health Care Online: The Role of Information Technologies*. U.S. Government Printing Office, Washington, D.C.

future, particularly in light of the additional genetic information that will become available as a result of advances such as those associated with the human genome project. Already, evidence exists to support claims that individuals experience discrimination by employers, insurers, and others based on the existence of genetic predispositions to particular ailments rather than on manifestations of such ailments.[34] Furthermore, even if individuals are not necessarily subject to economic discrimination as the result of such information, they may well wish to limit the dissemination or availability of information that might be embarrassing (e.g., a history of sexually transmitted diseases, treatment for depression, or a familial history of alcoholism).

Legislative Initiatives

In an attempt to improve protections for health information, a number of bills were introduced in the 104th Congress to address the use and disclosure of health information and to establish civil and criminal penalties for misuse of such information. These included the Medical Records Confidentiality Act of 1995 (S. 1360), Fair Health Information Practices Act of 1995 (H.R. 435), Medical Privacy in the Age of New Technologies Act of 1996 (H.R. 3482), and Health Insurance Portability and Accountability (HIPA) Act of 1996 (H.R. 3103). The Fair Information Practices Act was reintroduced into the 105th Congress in January 1997. Of these, only HIPA has been signed into law.

HIPA contains several provisions regarding health data standards and health information privacy. The purposes of these provisions are (1) to improve the efficiency and effectiveness of the health care delivery system by standardizing the electronic exchange of administrative and financial data and (2) to protect the confidentiality and security of transmitted health information.

Under HIPA, the Secretary of Health and Human Services is required to adopt standards by February 1998 providing for a unique health identifier for each individual, employer, health plan, and health care provider for use in the health care system. The Secretary is also required to adopt security standards that take into account (1) the technical capabilities of record systems used to maintain health information; (2) the costs of security measures; (3) the need for training persons who have access to health information; (4) the value of audit trails in computerized record systems;

---

[34]Billings, Paul R., Mel A. Kohn, Margaret de Cuevas, Jonathan Beckwith, Joseph S. Alper, and Marvin R. Natowicz. 1992. "Discrimination as a Consequence of Genetic Testing," *American Journal of Human Genetics* 50:476-482.

and (5) the needs and capabilities of small health care providers and rural health care providers.

HIPA requires that each person who maintains or transmits health information shall maintain reasonable and appropriate administrative, technical, and physical safeguards to ensure the integrity and confidentiality of the information; to protect against any reasonably anticipated threats or hazards to the security or integrity of the information and unauthorized uses or disclosures of the information; and to ensure that a health care clearinghouse, if it is part of a larger organization, has policies and security procedures that isolate its activities with respect to processing information in a manner that prevents unauthorized access to such information.

By August 1997, the Secretary is required to submit to Congress detailed recommendations on standards with respect to the privacy of individually identifiable health information. These recommendations must address the rights that should be guaranteed to an individual who is a subject of patient-identifiable health information, the procedures that should be established for the exercise of such rights, and the uses and disclosures that should be authorized or required. HIPA contains penalties ranging from $50,000 to $250,000 and 1 to 10 years in jail for wrongful disclosure of individually identifiable health information.

If legislation is not enacted by August 1997, the Secretary is required to promulgate final regulations containing such standards not later than 6 months after that date. In carrying out this section, the Secretary must consult with the National Committee on Vital and Health Statistics and the Attorney General.

The Health Insurance Portability and Accountability Act represents an important first step in better protection of health information. By mandating the promulgation of standards and regulations for security and privacy, the act begins to fill the void in existing legislation for protecting health information. It remains to be seen, however, how the act will be implemented and whether its standards and regulations will be enforced firmly. Without strong measures and ways of ensuring that they are implemented, patient health information may continue to remain vulnerable to potential misuse.

3
Privacy and Security Concerns Regarding Electronic Health Information

Concerns over the privacy and security of electronic health information fall into two general categories: (1) concerns about inappropriate releases of information from individual organizations and (2) concerns about the systemic flows of information throughout the health care and related industries. Inappropriate releases from organizations can result either from authorized users who intentionally or unintentionally access or disseminate information in violation of organizational policy or from outsiders who break into an organization's computer system. The second category—systemic concerns—refers to the open disclosure of patient-identifiable health information to parties that may act against the interests of the specific patient or may otherwise be perceived as invading a patient's privacy. These concerns arise from the many flows of data across the health care system, between and among providers, payers, and secondary users, with or without the patient's knowledge. These two categories of concerns are conceptually quite different and require different interventions or countermeasures.

CONCERNS REGARDING HEALTH INFORMATION HELD BY INDIVIDUAL ORGANIZATIONS

Electronic health records stored at individual organizations are vulnerable to internal or external agents that seek to violate directly the security and confidentiality policies of a specific organization (such agents are referred to as the "organizational threat" in this report). Internal

54

agents consist of authorized system users who abuse their privileges by accessing information for inappropriate reasons or uses, whether to view records of friends, neighbors, or coworkers or to leak information to the press. External agents consist of outsiders who are not authorized to use an information system or access its data, but who nevertheless attempt to access or manipulate data or to render the system inoperable. Health care organizations have long attempted to counter internal agents in their efforts to protect paper health records. They have less experience in protecting health information from technical attacks by outsiders because until recently, few health care organizations were connected to publicly accessible networks.

Scale of the Threat to Health Information Held by Individual Organizations

As yet, little evidence exists with which to gauge the vulnerability of electronic health information to outside attacks. The sites visited as part of this study reported no cases in which damaging intrusions by someone outside the site were detected,[1] and no mechanisms exist in the health care industry for reporting incidents. Nevertheless, computer break-ins are known to have occurred in the health care industry. In one case, the so-called "414" group broke into a machine at the National Cancer Institute in 1982,[2] although no damage was detected as a result of the intrusion.

Concerns over technical attacks by outsiders are rising in a number of other industry sectors and government. Commenting on a recent study by the Federal Bureau of Investigation and the Computer Security Institute (CSI), CSI Director Patrice Rapalus said, "The information age has already arrived, but most organizations are woefully unprepared . . . [making] it easier for perpetrators to steal, spy, or sabotage without being noticed and with little culpability if they are."[3] As a result of sampling 400 sites, the study further stated that 42 percent of the sites had experienced an intrusion or unauthorized use over the past year, 20 percent of the respondents did not know if their sites had been invaded, only 17

---

[1]One of the sites visited had detected the unauthorized use proprietary software by a summer student on an internal network, but no actual damage was detected. A few sites with protected connections to the Internet detected some inconsequential snooping at their points of entry, but did not consider intrusion by outsiders a significant problem .

[2]Marbach, William D. 1983. "Beware: Hackers at Play," *Newsweek*, September 5, p. 42-46.

[3]Power, Richard. 1996. "1996 CSI/FBI Computer Crime and Security Survey," *Computer Security Issues & Trends*, Vol. II, No. 2., Spring, p. 2.

percent of those suffering intrusions had notified authorities, and most respondents did not have a written policy for network intrusions. A recent estimate by the Defense Information Systems Agency indicated that Pentagon computers suffered 250,000 attacks by intruders in 1995; that this number is doubling each year; and that in about 65 percent of these attacks, intruders were able to gain entry to a computer network.[4] A RAND Corporation study of information warfare scenarios in 1995[5] suggests that terrorists using hacker technologies could wreak havoc in computer-based systems underlying 911 emergency telephone services, electric power distribution networks, banking and securities systems, train services, pipeline systems, information broadcast channels, and other parts of our information infrastructure.

While not specifically describing threats to health care organizations, these reports indicate the growing vulnerability of information systems connected to public infrastructure such as the Internet. As such, they suggest that the drive for increased use of electronic health information (e.g., digital patient records) linked together by modern networking technologies could expose sensitive health information to a variety of threats that will need to be appropriately addressed.

General Taxonomy of Organizational Threats

Organizational threats assume many forms, from employees who access data even though they have no legitimate need to know, to outside attackers who infiltrate an organization's information systems in order to steal data or destroy the system. Each type of threat is characterized by different motives, resources, avenues of accessing information systems, and technical capability. They therefore pose different degrees of risk to an organization and can be addressed with differing types of controls.

Factors Accounting for Differences Among Threats

Motive. Both economic and noneconomic factors can motivate attacks on health information. Patient health records have economic value to insurers, employers, and journalists. Noneconomic motives can include curiosity about the health status of friends, potential romantic involvements,

---

[4]General Accounting Office. 1996. *Information Security: Computer Attacks at Department of Defense Pose Increasing Risks.* General Accounting Office, Washington, D.C., May.

[5]Molander, Roger C., Andrew S. Riddile, and Peter A. Wilson. 1996. *Strategic Information Warfare: A New Face of War,* RAND Report MR-601. RAND Corporation, Santa Monica, Calif.

coworkers, or celebrities; clandestine observation of employees; and the desire to search the health records of parties involved in contentious interpersonal situations such as divorce or the breakup of intimate relationships.

Resources. With respect to resources available to them, potential attackers can range from individuals with modest financial and computing resources to well-funded and determined intelligence agencies and organized crime. In between lie medium and large organizations that have an economic interest in gathering health data. To date, the threat posed by intelligence agencies and organized crime has not surfaced in the health care arena.[6] The resources used in an attack against a health care organization are therefore those that would be available to an individual or a small group.

Initial Access. Initial access, the relationship of the attacker to the target data prior to the attacker's initiation of an assault on some stakeholder's system, has three elements:

1. *Site access.* The attacker either does or does not have the ability (or inclination) to enter the facility where data are accessed on a regular basis.
2. *System authorization.* The attacker either does or does not have authorization to use the information system in one way or another. System authorization is typically dependent on site access: a person without site access (either physical or electronic) is unlikely to have system authorization.
3. *Data authorization.* The attacker either does or does not have authorization to access the desired data. Data authorization is dependent on system authorization: a person without system authorization is unlikely to have data authorization.

These three elements of initial access can be combined in various ways to characterize a potential attacker. For example, an individual may have system authorization by virtue of being a financial clerk, not have data authorization for patient records, and have site access because he or she has a badge that allows movement freely about a hospital or clinic (Table 3.1). Site access is an important element when countermeasures are being considered.

---

[6]Whether such organizations are motivated to access patient health information improperly is not clear. Organized crime might be motivated by an interest in blackmailing an individual.

TABLE 3.1 Likely Combinations of Access Privileges in a Health Care Setting

Level of Access	Example
None	Outside attacker
Site only	Maintenance worker
Site and system	Worker in the billing department who has access to information systems but not to clinical information
Data and system	Vendor or consultant with remote access privileges
Site, system, and data	Care provider such as doctor or nurse

Technical Capability. The technical capability of an attacker is, in general, independent of the characteristics of access outlined above: an authorized user may be highly capable, and an unauthorized user may be computer illiterate. The technical capabilities of potential attackers can be characterized by three broad categories: *aspiring attackers, script runners,* and *accomplished attackers.*

Aspiring attackers are individuals with little or no computer expertise, but with ambitions and desires to learn more. They learn about attacks from popular literature, much of it published by organizations that cater to the survivalist and antiestablishment trade. The techniques they use are relatively unsophisticated and include the following:

• Researching the target site by reading open literature and scouting the location;
• Masquerading as an employee or other authorized individual to gain information or access;
• Guessing passwords, locating passwords written on calendars or elsewhere, or watching users enter their passwords;
• Searching trash bins for information on security practices and mechanisms; and
• Gaining entry to the desired location by gaining employment as a temporary employee, dressing as a custodial or professional staff member, or using some other method.

Script runners are an Internet phenomenon. These are individuals who obtain standard, scripted attacks and run them against information systems to which they desire entry. They generally have little or no knowledge of how the attacks work, do not care about learning more, and are unable to proceed further if the scripts fail. The current inventory of scripts operates primarily in standard Internet environments; given the rush of other vendors (e.g., Microsoft and IBM) to make their products Internet compatible, this level of technical capability will soon be able to be directed against all products using the Internet.

Accomplished attackers are the most formidable threat: they understand system vulnerabilities and are capable of adapting to situations where scripted attacks fail. For a health care organization, the worst-case future scenario is an accomplished attacker gaining entry via the Internet to an information system that allows access to patient health information.

The technical capability of attackers at each level in this hierarchy is constantly evolving and improving. Techniques that just a few years ago were the exclusive purview of accomplished attackers have moved to the script runner stage and will shortly be available to aspiring attackers. Mechanisms for countering these threats must therefore also evolve and improve, which implies a continuing intellectual and financial investment in security technology.

Levels of Threat to Information in Health Care Organizations

During its site visits, the committee discerned a number of distinct types of organizational threats described by different combinations of motive, resources, access, and technical capability. They are categorized here by levels numbered one through five (with five being the most sophisticated).

- *Threat 1: Insiders who make "innocent" mistakes and cause accidental disclosures.* Accidental disclosure of personal information—probably the most common source of breached privacy—happens in myriad ways, such as overheard conversations between care providers in the corridor or elevator, a laboratory technician's noticing test results for an acquaintance among laboratory tests being processed, information left on the screen of a computer in a nursing station so that a passerby can see it, misaddressed e-mail or fax messages, or misfiled and misclassified data.
- *Threat 2: Insiders who abuse their record access privileges.* Examples of this threat include individuals who have authorized access to health data (whether through on-site or off-site facilities) and who violate the trust associated with that access. Health care workers are subject to curiosity in accessing information they have neither the need nor the right to know. Although no overall statistics are available to indicate the scope of the problem, discussions with employees during site visits uncovered many cases in which health care workers have accessed information about the

health of fellow employees or family members out of concern for their well-being. There are reports of health care workers accessing health records to determine the possibility of sexually transmitted diseases in colleagues with whom they were having a relationship—or in people with whom former spouses were having relationships. Potentially embarrassing health information (e.g., psychiatric care episodes, substance abuse, physical abuse, abortions, HIV status, and sexually transmitted diseases) about politicians, entertainers, sports figures, and other prominent people regularly finds its way into the media.

• *Threat 3: Insiders who knowingly access information for spite or for profit.* This type of threat arises when an attacker has authorization to some part of the system but not to the desired data and through technical or other means gains unauthorized access to that data. An example is a billing clerk who exploits a system vulnerability to obtain access to data on a patient's medical condition. For example, the *London Sunday Times* reported in November 1995 that the contents of anyone's (electronic) health record in Great Britain could be purchased on the street for about £150 (or about $230).[7]

• *Threat 4: The unauthorized physical intruder.* In this case, the attacker has physical entry to points of data access but has no authorization for system use or the desired data. An example of this threat is an individual who puts on a lab coat and a fake badge, walks into a facility, and starts using a workstation or asking employees for health information.

• *Threat 5: Vengeful employees and outsiders, such as vindictive patients or intruders, who mount attacks to access unauthorized information, damage systems, and disrupt operations.* This is the pure technical threat—an attacker with no authorization and no physical access. An example is the intruder who breaks into a system from an external network and extracts patient records. Threat 5 is truly dangerous only when patient records are accessed regularly through an external network. It is clear that most providers are moving toward the use of networking and distributed computing technologies as they move toward electronic medical records. Threat 5 is therefore a latent problem on the horizon. The current reliance on paper records and the preoccupation of system managers with internal systems make threat 5 low in perceived importance and, so far, low in reported incidence. This situation is unlikely to last past the point at which internal systems are connected to external networks.

Threat 5 also encompasses "denial-of-service" attacks conducted electronically by outsiders. Such attacks are intended to render the attacked

---

[7]Rogers, L., and D. Leppard. 1995. "For Sale: Your Secret Medical Records for £150," *London Sunday Times,* November 26, pp. 1-2.

system useless for normal purposes. For example, an outside intruder may access a critical health information system not just to snoop on data but to insert a computer virus or Trojan horse that "crashes" the system at some later date or erases critical data files. Alternatively, an outsider could launch an e-mail attack in which a remote computer sends tens of thousands of e-mail messages in a very short time (e.g., an hour) to a given site, overwhelming the ability of the mail servers to process mail and rendering the system useless for ordinary e-mail purposes.

Countering Organizational Threats

There are two basic approaches to countering organizational threats to the privacy and security of electronic health information: deterrence and imposition of obstacles. Deterrence seeks to prevent violations of policy by imposing sanctions on violators; these sanctions may include dismissal, civil liability, or criminal prosecution. Obstacles are erected to prevent violations of policy by making them hard to achieve. Practical systems adopt a mixture of the two approaches; thus, in physical security one may install a reasonably strong lock (an obstacle) and an alarm system (representing deterrence, because apprehension in the act of breaking in carries criminal sanctions).

Deterrence assumes that individuals who constitute a threat can be identified and subjected to such sanctions. Technical support for deterrence centers on mechanisms for identifying users and auditing their actions. Obstacles are most often used in situations in which the threat cannot be identified or it is not practical to impose sanctions, such as in the protection of military or diplomatic information. Technical supports for imposition of obstacles include mechanisms for making a priori determinations of authorized use and then taking active steps to prevent unauthorized acts.

Three factors inhibit organizational adoption of obstacles: (1) the direct cost of the mechanisms, such as access control tokens, and cryptographic devices; (2) the indirect cost of decreased efficiency and morale (e.g., the "hassle factor" of an additional inconvenience); and (3) the possibility that an obstacle may prevent necessary, legitimate access or use of data (e.g., in an emergency or some other situation not anticipated by the mechanism's designer). Deterrence mechanisms also entail costs, but these costs tend to be more indirect (e.g., personnel costs in educating users about the existence of penalties for abusing access privileges).

Developing Appropriate Countermeasures

Specific countermeasures have to be developed for each of the five threats outlined above. Health care organizations must therefore assess their information systems to determine the types of threats to which they are most vulnerable and must then implement the necessary organizational and technical mechanisms. Although the precise implementation will vary from one institution to another, some general rules of thumb apply across organizations (Table 3.2). Specific ways of implementing the types of mechanisms identified are outlined in Chapters 4 and 5.

Threat 1 can best be countered by organizational mechanisms that detect and deter abuses. More sophisticated technology per se can do little to prevent this kind of disclosure. Simple procedural measures appear to be most appropriate—for example, reminders about behavioral codes, confirmation of actions that might route or access information erroneously, or screen savers and automatic log-outs to prevent access to unattended displays. Chapter 4 examines the possibility of extending these procedures by maintaining patient anonymity through the use of coded patient identifiers (pseudonyms) in most of the care process.

The principal countermeasure for threat 2 is deterrence: appeals to ethics, education about what constitutes fair practice, and the imposition of sanctions after an incident occurs. Technology can also play a role in controlling inappropriate access to patient information. Strong user authentication, based on cryptographic techniques, can effectively control access to health information networks and computer systems—at least to the extent that system users protect their identifying data and make appropriate use of the information they are authorized to access. The use of encryption can place significant obstacles in the way of potential abusers, requiring them to obtain special data (keys) to make patient information legible. Properly analyzed audit records of accesses are another powerful tool to deter abuse.

A combination of obstacles and deterrence is necessary to counter threat 3. These include reasonable obstacles to prevent unauthorized access without interfering with authorized use and the deterrence steps used against threat 2. Audit trails are particularly effective at deterring this type of threat.

The countermeasures for threat 4 rely heavily on deterrence, supplemented with strong technical obstacles. Attackers run the risk of immediate identification and apprehension and have the potential of leaving physical evidence of intrusion (e.g., surveillance tapes) that can be used in prosecution. The obstacles that can be placed in the way of threat 4 include both technical security measures such as strong identification and authentication mechanisms and physical security measures such as requiring badges, and challenging strangers.

Countermeasures against threat 5 are based purely on the obstacle approach. In this case, the threat is not readily identifiable; its physical

TABLE 3.2 Types of Threat to Health Information Held by Health Care Organizations and Possible Countermeasures

Type	System Authorization	Data Authorization	Site Access	Threat	Countermeasure
1	Yes	Yes	Yes	Mistakes	Organizational and simple technical mechanisms
2	Yes	Yes	n/a	Improper use of access privileges	Organizational and technical mechanisms such as authentication and auditing
3	Yes	No	n/a	Unauthorized use for spite or profit	Organizaitonal and technical mechanisms such as authentication and auditing
4	No	No	Yes	Unauthorized physical intrusion	Physical security and technical mechanisms such as authentication and access controls
5	No	No	No	Technical break-in	Technical mechanisms such as authentication, access controls, and cryptography

location is not easily determined; and the threat may not be subject to any credible administrative, civil, or criminal sanctions (e.g., an intruder based overseas). Technological obstacles to intruders include the use of firewalls to isolate internal and external networks and strong encryption-based authentication and authorization technologies to prevent intruders from masquerading as legitimate users. However, the effectiveness of technological obstacles can be ensured only when network connections between the health information system and the outside world are restricted administratively to passing nonsensitive data (e.g., e-mail unrelated to patient care, access to the World Wide Web for research data). If external network connections are used for both sensitive and nonsensitive data, then the technical countermeasures required to guarantee security may well push the state of the art,[8] to say nothing of exceeding the state of practice observed in the site visits. Furthermore, for some types of attack, there are no known obstacles at all; for example, denial-of-service attacks based on exhaustion of resources are very hard to defend against, especially when timeliness of response is an issue, although defenses against denial-of-service attacks can sometimes be created on an ad hoc basis. This is not to say that technical countermeasures are useless (indeed, the focus of Chapter 4 is on technical countermeasures that can be deployed to useful effect). Nevertheless, technical countermeasures cannot be viewed as a cure-all for security problems.

Observations on Countering Organizational Threats

Obstacles such as encryption and authentication are the only effective ways to counter organizational threats against systems that have an Internet interface because there are minimal, if any, accountability mechanisms in effect on the Internet. In addition, the Internet spans multiple legal and national jurisdictions. (The same holds true—to a lesser degree—for systems with any kind of "dial-in" interface.) As a consequence, extensive use of the Internet to access or transfer health record data will carry with it a significant and growing risk from organizational threats to the security and privacy of the data unless steps are taken to mitigate this risk; these steps are the focus of Chapter 4 and Chapter 6 . The largest portion of these risks will not be mitigated until ways are developed of holding Internet users accountable for their actions and agreements are in place across multiple legal and national jurisdictions to impose sanctions for violations of the security and privacy of health information.

Until these steps are taken, the use of the Internet for the access and

---

[8]Constance, Paul. 1996. "Multi-level Security—Not Now," *Government Computer News*, July 15, p. 60.

transfer of health information will have to be limited to those tasks that convenient obstacle-based security mechanisms can support; the culture of stakeholders will have to change to accommodate the extra load of mechanisms that are more difficult to use; or the aforementioned risks will have to be assumed by the health care system.

Provided that adequate obstacle-based security mechanisms exist at the Internet interface (e.g., by use of a firewall), a deterrence-based approach that allows relatively free internal access can be adopted without excessive risk. Countering organizational threats by erecting technical obstacles to access is not, in general, compatible with the efficient and effective operation of systems used by providers. The time pressures on providers do not permit the level of security-driven interaction that such mechanisms require, and the risk that an obstacle-based mechanism will deny legitimate access to data in an emergency (with the consequent liability) is inherent in such mechanisms. An important enabling mechanism for such an approach is an identification and authentication mechanism that has adequate strength and is acceptable to all classes of users.

SYSTEMIC CONCERNS ABOUT HEALTH INFORMATION

Systemic concerns about the privacy of patient-specific health information are generally rooted in the use of such information in a manner that acts against the interests of the individual patient involved. These interests may involve specific identifiable adverse consequences such as increased difficulty in obtaining employment or insurance or less tangible ones such as personal embarrassment or discomfort. In order to understand how public concerns about such use arise, it is helpful first to examine the exchanges of health information throughout the health care system.

Uses and Flows of Health Information

Health information—both paper and electronic—is used for many purposes by a variety of individuals and organizations within and outside the health care industry (Table 3.3). Primary users include physicians, clinics, and hospitals that provide care to patients. Secondary users employ health information for a variety of societal, business, and government purposes other than providing care.[9] They include organizations that pay for health care benefits, such as traditional insurance companies, managed care providers, or government programs like Medicare and

---

[9]*Consumer Reports.* 1994. "Who's Reading Your Medical Records?," October, pp. 628-632.

TABLE 3.3 Typical Users and Uses of Health Information

User	Purpose	Patient Identifiable?
Patient	• To provide historical information to primary care physician • To authenticate health insurance coverage and responsibility for paying health care claims • To complete application for life insurance	Yes
Primary care physician	• To assess patient's medical needs • To document patient's medical needs for continuity of care • To develop an appropriate treatment plan • To prescribe diagnostic tests, order treatment, etc. • To work with patient to ensure success of treatment plan • To work with other physicians as necessary to provide treatment • To maintain ongoing record of services provided to patient • To bill either patient or health insurance company for services provided to patient	Yes
Health insurance company	• To process health care claims to reimburse provider of services • To approve consultation requests by primary care physician	Yes
Clinical laboratory	• To process and analyze patient's specimen • To report results of analysis to patient's primary care physician • To maintain record of results of analysis • To bill patient, primary care physician, or health insurance company for services provided	Yes
Local retail pharmacy	• To fill prescription for treatment of patient's condition • To bill patient's pharmacy benefit program for medication	Yes
Pharmacy benefits manager	• To process claim for medications provided to patient by local pharmacy • To monitor prescription and suggest generic substitutes to patient's physician • To perform utilization review of patient's physician	Yes

TABLE 3.3   Continued

User	Purpose	Patient Identifiable?
Consulting physician	• To assess patient's medical needs • To document patient's medical needs for continuity of care • To develop an appropriate treatment plan • To prescribe diagnostic tests, order treatment, etc. • To work with patient to ensure success of treatment plan • To work with primary care physician as necessary to provide treatment • To maintain ongoing record of services provided to patient • To bill either patient or health insurance company for services provided to patient	Yes
Local hospital	• To provide care to patient as directed by patient's primary care physician • To maintain ongoing record of services provided to patient • To bill either patient or health insurance company for services provided to patient • To complete and send birth certificates to state's office of vital statistics	Yes
State bureau of vital statistics	• To record birth of patient's baby in state registry • To initiate an immunization record	Yes; baby also identifiable
Accrediting organization	• To review local hospital's operations • To recommend improvement in operations based on review of patient records • To accredit local hospital for meeting both operational and quality standards	Yes
Employer	• To request claims data on employees • To review claims data to identify ways to reduce claims • To adjust benefits package based on review of data	Possibly
Life insurance company	• To process patient's application for life insurance • To request medical examination as a prerequisite for life insurance	Yes

continued on next page

TABLE 3.3   Continued

User	Purpose	Patient Identifiable?
	• To contact Medical Insurance Bureau (MIB) for patient's prior medical history so as to assess risk • To grant life insurance to patient • To report relevant information to MIB	
Medical Information Bureau	• To retain health information on individuals requesting life insurance • To provide health information on individuals applying for insurance from MIB members, to reduce fraud	Yes
Managed care company	• To process health care claims • To evaluate consultation requests by primary care physician • To assess quality and appropriateness of care	Yes
Attorney	• To understand standard of practice by specialists treating specific ailments • To request data demonstrating adherence to standard of practice • To analyze data demonstrating adherence to standard of practice	No
State public health and family physician	• To perform metabolic screening on newborns through blood tests	Yes; baby also identifiable
State agency collecting hospital discharge data	• To analyze health services utilization and hospital cost and effectiveness of health care delivery	Yes; baby also identifiable
Medical researcher	• To research the appropriateness and effects of a patient's medication	No

Medicaid. As part of their management functions, these payer organizations also conduct analyses of the quality of health care delivered by provider organizations and its relative costs. Other secondary users include medical and social science researchers, rehabilitation and social welfare programs, public health services, pharmaceutical companies, marketing firms, the judicial system, and the media. They use health information for purposes such as researching the costs and benefits of alternative treatment plans, determining eligibility for social programs, understanding state and local health needs, news reporting, and targeting possible markets for new or existing products. Marketing firms and vendors of health-related products also obtain health information that will help them target particular types of patients for direct marketing.[10]

The types of information collected by primary and secondary users vary greatly across individual organizations. Exchanges of data among these organizations are highly complex and dynamic. Rather than attempting to enumerate every possible flow, the discussion below traces the records of a hypothetical, but typical, patient named Alice. Alice's story is a representative, although by no means comprehensive, description of how health records are shared between organizations and individuals.

Alice's Medical Records

Alice is in her late twenties, married, and employed by a small company. Bob, her husband, is employed by a large firm. Bob's company offers its employees a choice of three health benefit plans: (1) a health maintenance organization (HMO) that operates its own clinics and pharmacies and permits referrals to outside physicians only under strict guidelines; (2) a preferred provider organization (PPO) that provides pharmacy benefits and reimburses charges from participating physicians at a higher rate than those from nonparticipating physicians, but allowing patients to choose physicians freely; and (3) a conventional indemnity insurance program in which all charges are reimbursed at the same rate after an annual deductible is met, with supplementary major health insurance to cover extraordinary expenses. Differences in the ways their health records may be stored and controlled are not outlined in the program descriptions, and Alice and Bob do not consider this factor in their decision. Hoping to save money but preserve choice of physicians, Bob and Alice choose the PPO option. Bob's employer is self-insured—an increasingly popular strategy for many large employers—though this fact is not stated openly during the enrollment process.

When they set up housekeeping in their current location, Alice and Bob consult friends, colleagues, and local sources of information to find

---

[10]Some states sell driver's license records, complete with height, weight, full name, and address, and allow focused marketing based on any of these characteristics. Demographic information purchased from a particular type of organization, such as an AIDS clinic, a maternal care center, or a wellness program can also help target individuals for specific marketing campaigns.

primary care providers. On her first visit to a prospective primary physician, who is a member of a small group practice, Alice is asked to fill out a medical history form and specify how she will pay for her care in the future. She indicates that she will use the health insurance benefits available to her through her husband's job. Since Alice specifies that some of her charges will be covered by a party other than herself, she is also given a form to sign that would authorize the physician's office to send information to the insurer for payment of claims. This release covers all future visits Alice makes to this practice.

Alice's initial visit is satisfactory, and she decides to use this physician as her primary care provider. Records for her initial examination are recorded on paper and held in the physician's office. Blood samples taken from her during the visit, however, are sent to an outside laboratory for analysis. Automated analysis equipment records the laboratory results and prints a paper copy that is returned to the physician; the laboratory bills Alice for the service. The laboratory also retains a record of the test and of Alice's identity. Through the third-party administrator used by Bob's firm to manage health care benefits, Bob's firm receives a claim from Alice for the office visit and the blood test, and approves payment.

The following year, Alice's annual checkup reveals hypertension, and blood tests show mild anemia. The physician prescribes two medications, and Alice fills the prescriptions at a local pharmacy. The pharmacy's charges are reimbursed through a pharmacy benefits program connected with the health insurance option selected by Bob. The pharmacy records Alice's name and address, reads her pharmacy benefits card, notifies the benefits program, and is reimbursed. Parts of Alice's health record now reside with the retail pharmacy and the pharmacy benefits provider, as well as her care provider.

When Alice becomes pregnant, she develops a condition that her primary care provider wishes to discuss with another physician outside the group. She requests Alice's permission to release information to the consulting physician, since Alice may wish a second opinion, and Alice will pay for part of the cost. Acting in accordance with the rules specified by Bob's firm, the third-party administrator approves both the consultation and part of the consultant's fee. The primary care provider trusts the consultant to keep information in Alice's record confidential.

The child is delivered at a local hospital used by the group practice. Prior to Alice's admission, she provides evidence of her ability to pay by showing her insurance card, and she signs a form authorizing the hospital to release to paying parties any data from this admission required for payment. The hospital performs a variety of tests and procedures during Alice's stay and creates a related set of records, some automated and some on paper. The child's birth is recorded with the state, which also opens an immunization record for the child.

Subsequently, the hospital is visited by an accrediting body, which, as a routine part of its investigation, checks on the record-keeping procedures at the hospital. As it happens, Alice's records are among those reviewed, but the accreditors do not remove them from the hospital or make any copies. They simply check the records for accuracy and completeness and to ensure that they are stored in compliance with accrediting procedures.

Bob's company, feeling competitive pressures, considers ways to save money and increase productivity. Improving employees' health seems to be a positive step, since it may both decrease claims and improve performance. Since Bob's company is self-insuring, it asks the third-party administrator to provide it with claims information pertaining to its employees. Though reluctant to share patient-identifiable information because of concerns over privacy, the third-party administrator has no legal basis on which to refuse the request and, to maintain good relations with its client, provides the information to Bob's employer.[11] Since her claims are paid by Bob's company, Alice's record, as well as Bob's, is also forwarded. Alice's company, under similar pressure, initiates a company clinic on-site and a "wellness" program. Although she continues to be insured by Bob's company, Alice uses the clinic occasionally and, on her first visit, provides the clinic with her history, including a list of medications she is taking.

After the birth of their child, Bob and Alice realize that they need life insurance. Both of their companies provide some group coverage, but it is inadequate for their needs. Alice applies for coverage with a large, respected firm, which will provide the coverage she wants if she passes a physical examination. The life insurance company will pay for the examination, but she must sign a release permitting the results of the examination to be forwarded to the Medical Information Bureau (MIB). The life insurance company decides to accept the risk of insuring her but forwards the hypertension results to the MIB in accordance with the industry's practices because her hypertension, although under control, may potentially affect her longevity.

The group practice Alice uses is purchased by a managed care firm, which installs its automated records program. Results of Alice's office visits are now stored on a local computer system. The managed care firm, facing the same competitive pressures as Bob's company, periodically

---

[11] Not all insurers will provide such information to self-insured clients, but others report that they do because they have no legal basis on which to refuse.

reviews records from each of its many groups to ensure both the quality and the appropriateness of the care provided.

The managed care firm denies a request from another patient within the practice to consult a specialist for a condition similar to the one for which Alice was treated. The patient subsequently sues the practice, and her lawyers request disclosure of records from similar cases within the practice. The court grants a subpoena for the records involved, including Alice's, and the practice is compelled to provide copies of the records to lawyers. Alice's name is removed from the record.

A researcher wants to investigate the long-term effects of the hypertension medication Alice has been taking. He gets a federal grant to support the study and gains approval of his organization's institutional review board. He then writes to hospitals and physicians to request access to their records. Alice's physician contacts Alice and several other patients to ask if they are willing to participate in the study. Alice agrees and signs a consent form granting her physician permission to provide her records to the researcher for purposes of this study, but she insists that her identity not be revealed. The records are provided as requested, but with the name, address, and Social Security number fields scrambled in such a way as to allow Alice's records to be linked without divulging her identity.

At this point, parts of Alice's health record are held by a wide variety of organizations: her primary care physician's practice, a clinical laboratory, the local pharmacy, the pharmacy benefits provider, the practice of the consulting physician, the local hospital, the state bureau of vital statistics, the hospital accrediting agency, her husband's employer, her life insurance company, the Medical Information Bureau, the outcomes researcher, and various lawyers (Figure 3.1). Most of these organizations have information that specifically identifies Alice. She has explicitly consented to grant access to some of these holders; she is aware of others to whom she has not granted access; of others, she may be entirely unaware. If Alice and Bob had chosen a different health plan, the flows might differ. A comprehensive HMO, providing medical, hospital, and pharmacy service, might have more flows within it and fewer outside organizations, for example.

Government Collection of Health Data

If Alice were an impoverished single parent receiving government benefits, additional flows of data would involve state and federal social services agencies. The federal government collects data for reimbursement of care provided under Medicare and Medicaid, but states also collect large amounts of patient-identifiable information for their own pur-

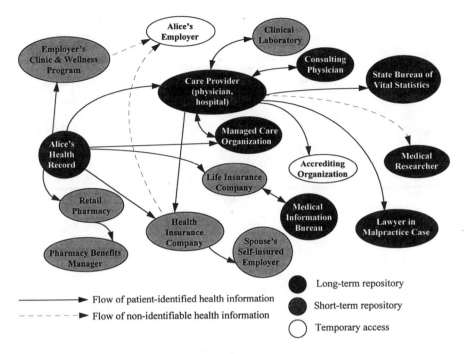

FIGURE 3.1   Flows of Alice's health information.

poses. State health agencies can provide services and collect identifiable data about patients just as providers in private health care entities would. Functioning as providers, they would release identifiable data with patient consent to insurers and other providers depending on the need to know. State health agencies collect data for the purposes of analyzing and disseminating information on health status, personal health problems, population groups at risk, availability and quality of services, and health resource availability.[12] The categories of data collected are dependent on the services and functions each health department has within its authority. Environmental services, Medicaid, professional and facility licensing, and alcohol and drug abuse or mental health services are not located consistently in all state health departments across the country.

State health departments generally collect patient-identifiable data

---

[12] For a review and analysis of state laws that regulate the acquisition, storage, and use of public health data, see Gostin, Lawrence O., Zita Lazzarini, Verla S. Neslund, and Michael T. Osterholm, 1996, "The Public Health Information Infrastructure: A National Review of the Law on Health Information Privacy," *Journal of the American Medical Association* 275(24):1921-1927.

related to health service utilization and costs, personal health status and risk (health surveillance data), alcohol and drug abuse services, and mental health services, among other categories. The types of data systems related to each of these categories can be extensive (Table 3.4).

Databases created for these purposes generally have a designated steward who is responsible for managing the protection and the uses of the data. These types of data are released in an identifiable form only in select situations: (1) research purposes for which there has been an approved human subjects review and a data-sharing agreement that outlines restrictions on the use of data, destruction of data at the end of research, and the penalties for violating the agreement; and (2) the investigation of a reportable disease or condition for the purposes of protecting the public's health. In the latter case, identifiable data are released to specially authorized public health investigators or private physicians who are responsible for care of the person believed to have a reportable condition or disease (e.g., measles, sexually transmitted disease, tuberculosis, birth defect, cancer). The steward of the database determines which staff members are allowed to access identifiable data for the purposes of analyzing them. Finally, state laws include penalties that prohibit improper release of data by a state government employee.

Risks Created by Systemic Flows of Health Information

As Alice's story shows, the types of organizations that collect, process, and store health information include not only other members of health care provider teams, such as referral providers, nurses, and laboratory technicians, but also groups such as insurance companies and third-party payers, utilization and outcomes assessment groups, public health and disease registry groups, clinical research groups, and a growing health information services industry. These various organizations have historically developed separate policies with regard to the protection of information in these records. These separate policies reflect the different perceptions of individual stakeholders regarding the proper trade-off between Alice's privacy interests and their use of the data. Although these policies are not always formalized or documented, a consensus among the members of each stakeholder group can generally be discerned.

Such consensus typically does not exist between different groups of stakeholders (e.g., providers and insurers) or between managed care organizations and self-insured employers. A collection of health insurance executives is likely to agree regarding the bounds of legitimate access within their own business sector, as is a collection of physicians, but the two definitions of legitimate access are likely to differ significantly from one another. As a result, the movement of data around a network of

TABLE 3.4 Typical Health Information Collected by State Health Departments

Data Set	Content
Hospital discharge data	Information on all patients discharged from acute care hospitals; systems track morbidity, hospital use and costs, and the distribution and utilization of services
Clinic visit records	Information on family planning services utilization
Genetics clinics reports	Summary statistics on services and volumes of contracted genetic counseling clinics
Adult immunization survey	Information on vaccination status of adults in schools and adults in health care facilities
Child immunization tracking	Information on individual childhood immunizations and rates
AIDS reporting system	Information on all reported Class IV AIDS cases; used for disease surveillance and trend analysis
Behavioral risk factor surveillance system	Yearly telephone survey on health-related behaviors of a sample of individuals 18 and older, used to develop statewide prevalence estimates to target preventive health services to counties, age groups, and so on
Birth certificate file	Information on all births occurring in a particular state; used to monitor trends in population fertility and maternal and child morbidity, to establish legal residence, and to assist in epidemiological analyses
Birth events records file	Linkage of records from the Hospital Abstract System
Cancer registries	Documentation of statewide incidences of cancer from hospital tumor registries and laboratory data
Birth certificate file and infant file	Information from studies on prenatal care and outcomes studies
Death certificate file	Information on all deaths occurring in a particular state; used to monitor trends in mortality, establish legal benefits, and assist in epidemiological analyses

continued on next page

TABLE 3.4 Continued

Data Set	Content
Fetal death file	Information on all fetal deaths (gestation periods of 20 weeks or more)
Newborn screening data	Information on laboratory tests for hemoglobinopathies, which are performed on all newborns delivered in hospitals in the state; used for early identification and treatment of these disorders
Long-term care facility influenza and pneumococcal survey data	Information on immunization status for residents and staff of long-term care facility
Rash data	Information on new cases of measles and vaccination status of those cases
Monitoring system for adverse events following immunization	Tracking of suspected events following immunization; used to initiate follow-up action if needed
Occupational mortality data	Information on occupation-related mortality and effects of occupational exposures on natality
Reportable diseases and conditions	Information of occurrences of diseases (used for disease surveillance) and conditions
Sexually transmitted disease morbidity and epidemiological reports	Information on morbidity and epidemiological investigations and follow-up actions for individuals or partners testing positive for sexually transmitted diseases
Tuberculosis case registry and contacts	Information on management of individual cases of persons with tuberculosis and individuals exposed to tuberculosis and their follow-up and treatment
Women, infants and children information set	Minimum information required by U.S. Department of Agriculture to certify clients for Women, Infants, and Children Supplemental Food Program
Child abuse and neglect data	Information on child abuse or neglect referrals, subsequent investigations, and responses to referrals and investigations

SOURCE: Washington State Department of Health, 1996: personal communication (October).

stakeholders (movement that often occurs without the consent that can be effectively withheld by the patient or primary provider) is not governed by any network-wide policy. Rather, data are treated in accordance with a variety of local policies that may or may not be consistent with the patient's understanding when signing a form that authorizes initial release of the information. Individual organizations often have strong business incentives to protect health information from other parties because they regard such information as having significant business value; nevertheless, almost all of the sites that the committee visited during the course of this study expressed serious concerns about potential harm to patient interests resulting from unrestrained use of patient information by organizations not involved in the provision of care.

Without industry-wide standards or regulations governing the uses of health information by primary and secondary users, the information can—and sometimes is—employed for purposes that violate patient privacy or are detrimental to the interests of the patient. One example of the kinds of harm that can befall patients is outlined in a recent case study[13] that describes the results of a survey in which 206 respondents reported discrimination as a result of access to genetic information. Such discrimination resulted in loss of employment, loss of insurance coverage, or ineligibility for insurance. The cases were screened carefully to identify those in which discrimination was based on the future potential for disease rather than existing manifestations of a particular malady (i.e., the patients exhibited no phenotypic evidence of disease, only a predisposition to a future occurrence of treatable diseases such as hemochromatosis, phenylketonuria, muco-polysaccharidoses, and Huntington's disease).

A second example of harm is illustrated by the case of a pharmaceutical company that acquired a drug reimbursement service or pharmaceutical benefits manager (PBM). The PBM used information in its database in an attempt to convince physicians to prescribe drugs manufactured by the pharmaceutical company. In a March 1996 consent decree filed in Minnesota and joined by 17 other states,[14] one such firm agreed to stop interfering in the prescription of medications from other manufacturers when it assessed patients' eligibility for coverage. Although no direct financial or physical harm befell patients in this case, their privacy interests were compromised when confidential information about them was

---

[13]Geller, L.N., J.S. Alper, P.R. Billings, C.I. Barash, J. Beckwith, and M. Natowicz. 1996. "Individual, Family, and Societal Dimensions of Genetic Discrimination: A Case Study Analysis," *Science and Engineering Ethics* 2(1):71-88.

[14]*PRNewswire.* 1996. "Minnesota Takes the Lead on Agreement to Protect 41 Million Americans," October 25; available on-line at www.epic.org/privacy/medical/merck.txt.

furnished to individuals (pharmacists) who were unconnected with the conduct or quality of their care.

These examples clearly suggest that the interests of patients may not be well served by wide dissemination of health care information. If Alice had developed an expensive, chronic condition as a complication of her pregnancy, Bob's self-insured employer could be made aware of that fact through its review of billing data (which contain detailed diagnostic codes) and could use such information to influence a decision about Bob's continued employment. Managers in Bob's company might well argue that Bob's high health insurance bills make him too expensive to keep on the payroll. In a recent survey of Fortune 500 corporations, 35 percent responded that they use individual health records in making employment-related decisions.[15] One in ten companies does not inform employees of this practice. An earlier survey indicated that 50 percent of the companies used health records in making employment-related decisions and that 19 percent did not inform employees of such use.[16] It is not clear from these studies *how* employers are using the data; there may be cases in which the information is used to benefit the employee,[17] but it can be argued that such decisions should be made by the employee. Furthermore, no legal standard prevents Bob's old employer from discussing Alice's condition with a potential new employer or prevents some entrepreneur from establishing a clearinghouse of data on employees with high insurance costs.

Universal Patient Identifiers

Concerns about the systemic sharing of electronic health information are linked to efforts to establish a universal patient identifier for indexing patient records throughout the U.S. health care system. The Health Insurance Portability and Accountability Act of 1996 directs the Secretary of Health and Human Services to promulgate a standard for such an identifier by February 1998. The goals of this initiative are multiple and include improving the quality of care by allowing providers to more easily locate patient records, facilitating health services research, and simplifying the administrative aspects of managing and paying for care. Optimal health

---

[15]Linowes, David F. 1996. "A Research Survey of Privacy in the Workplace," an unpublished white paper available from the University of Illinois at Urbana-Champaign.

[16]Linowes, David F. 1989. *Privacy in America: Is Your Private Life in the Public Eye?* University of Illinois Press, Urbana, Ill., p. 42.

[17]For example, the employer may shift a pregnant worker out of a hazardous environment.

care often depends on the availability of a complete medical record,[18] and health outcomes research depends on the ability to undertake longitudinal studies on individuals (although not necessarily studies that are linked to the identities of these individuals). Detecting fraud may be possible only when abuse is revealed through unusual patterns of health care usage (linked through individual patient records).

Large, integrated delivery systems and managed care programs routinely assign patients identifiers for use within their health care systems without generating much controversy.[19] What generates the largest amount of controversy is the prospect that a universal identifier will facilitate attempts to link information within and across much larger boundaries. For example, the idea of using the Social Security number (SSN) as a universal health identifier raises concerns not only that all medical data associated with a given individual can be linked, but also that an individual's medical data could be linked with financial data, purchasing habit data, family details, and other items of information—many of which are already indexed by the SSN—to create a personally identifiable, interlinked record containing sensitive information. The use of *any* single number as a universal identifier could expand beyond its initial intent and become widespread in other domains, just as use of the SSN expanded well beyond the realm of identifying Social Security records.[20]

Adoption of a universal patient identifier would raise concerns about its use to link large numbers of personal data transactions in two distinct areas:

1. *Discrimination:* Sensitive or adverse information may be used against an individual's economic interests in some way. For example, an employer may refuse to hire or promote an individual with a long and expensive history of medical claims (or with the prospect of expensive or chronic medical problems in the future based on genetics or family history).

2. *Loss of privacy:* Many individuals have medical conditions that they might wish to keep private (e.g., a history of sexually transmitted diseases or treatment for depression). Even if an individual is not subject

---

[18]It is advantageous for a patient in the emergency room or one who is being treated for substance abuse to have medical data linked so that care providers can make clinically informed decisions regarding care.

[19]If health care moves to a more integrated service model in which large megaorganizations are responsible for more dimensions of care and an individual has less choice in selecting the organization with which he or she will interact, controversy may yet develop.

[20]Szolovits, Peter, and Isaac Kohane. 1994. "Against Universal Health-care Identifiers," *Journal of the American Medical Informatics Association* 1:316-319.

to economic discrimination as the result of such a past, he or she may well wish to limit the dissemination or availability of such information.

Mitigating the impact of such concerns is generally a matter of public policy. Health care enterprises and others with access to health care information can decide voluntarily to refrain from using a universal health identifier in particular ways, or mandatory mechanisms can be put in place by legislation. Legislative approaches might choose to prohibit discrimination in employment on the basis of patient information or prohibit the dissemination of patient information to employers. Nevertheless, it may be possible to design an identification and linking scheme that can satisfy the needs of the health care industry without jeopardizing patient privacy or that can help enforce any policy framework established for protecting privacy. For example, it may be possible to design a system that does not rely on a single number. Chapter 4 outlines some approaches for identifying and linking records. Chapter 6 contains the committee's judgments on these issues. The chapters include recommendations for extensive education of the public about threats to the privacy of health care information and criteria for ensuring that the development of any universal patient identifier explicitly recognizes its potential effects on privacy. They also include recommendations for the passage of legislation setting down the principles by which trustees of health care information are limited in its collection, use, and disposal and are responsible for disclosure of accesses to it. Finally, they include the development of technologies that control the integrity of, access to, and accountability for uses of health care information across all stakeholders.

Conclusions Regarding Systemic Concerns

Patient-identifiable health information has business value to organizations such as insurers, employers, providers, and drug companies. This value leads to organizational pressure to disseminate and use the data for purposes other than those for which they were collected. Individual patients are at a disadvantage in resisting this pressure because of the imbalance of power between them and these organizations.

Systemic concerns arise from deep differences among stakeholders as to what constitutes fair information practice. Every stakeholder that receives data about a patient has an argument to support its claims about a bona fide need for patient information. No consensus exists across society regarding the legitimacy of these needs and against which they can be independently assessed. Nor does consensus exist regarding the uses made of such information. This lack of consensus differentiates the security problem in the health care field from that of the military or financial communities, for example, where a general consensus on information policy exists. As a consequence, security technology and practices from these other communities should be adopted only with great care.

Systemic concerns are exacerbated by technology, because computer networking permits rapid, large-scale, and unobserved access to data for uses never intended when the patient gave primary permission for the data to be recorded. To date, technological deterrents and obstacles play almost no role in controlling secondary use of patient information (i.e., use by nonprovider parties). Once the information leaves the hands of the health care provider, it is stored off-site with the secondary user, and access controls are at the discretion of that user site.

Systemic concerns will be reduced only by public policy decisions that influence the behavior of stakeholders regarding data privacy and security. These public policy decisions are necessary to rationalize the relationships among the various stakeholders (e.g., to spell out the acceptable uses of health care information by nonproviders and providers alike) and to reduce the incentives for wholesale release of patient information. Put differently, public policy must add up to a comprehensive whole that covers the entire network of use, including both primary and secondary uses of data. Because there is no consensus across society about what is acceptable, public policy in this area is difficult to make, but until such policy is in place, there is a progressive danger that care will be affected by patients' reluctance to confide in providers.

Systemic concerns are linked to development of a universal patient identifier, which, depending on its format, could facilitate the linking of patient-identifiable health information with other types of personal information. Although addressing this problem is largely a matter of public policy, judicious design of the method used to link patient records may help mitigate some privacy concerns and help enforce any policy framework established for protecting privacy.

4

Technical Approaches to Protecting Electronic Health Information

Technological security tools are essential components of modern distributed health care information systems. At the highest level, they serve five key functions:[1]

1. *Availability*—ensuring that accurate and up-to-date information is available when needed at appropriate places;
2. *Accountability*—helping to ensure that health care providers are responsible for their access to and use of information, based on a legitimate need and right to know;
3. *Perimeter identification*—knowing and controlling the boundaries of trusted access to the information system, both physically and logically;
4. *Controlling access*—enabling access for health care providers only to information essential to the performance of their jobs and limiting the real or perceived temptation to access information beyond a legitimate need; and
5. *Comprehensibility and control*—ensuring that record owners, data stewards, and patients understand and have effective control over appropriate aspects of information privacy and access.

Health care organizations evaluate security technologies in terms both

---

[1]Note that these functions—aimed at improving system security—are conceptually different from those that would be required by the work of a database administrator or a network manager.

of their functional benefits for protecting patient privacy and their costs: the cost of impeding or preventing clinicians from accessing information relevant to their decision making; the cost of purchasing and integrating them into the information system environment; the cost of ongoing management, operations, and maintenance of the evolving information system; the cost of user frustration with suboptimal interfaces and procedures; and the cost of user time lost in satisfying security requirements. They must also attempt to implement a *balanced* approach to protecting against threats to information security and the risks posed by violations. For example, if there are two equally likely and costly threats—e.g., power outages and insiders divulging information—resources should be allocated to protect approximately equally against these threats.[2]

Individual technologies vary widely in terms of these cost-benefit characteristics, and as new technologies are developed and reduced to commercial practice, their characteristics change with time. System managers must choose a set of technological interventions that provide effective protection against perceived threats to system security but impose acceptable overall costs. This choice is difficult at best and requires ongoing updates of threat models; evaluations of technologies; reconsideration of integration and operation strategies; and education of management, systems staff, and users. This trade-off almost never includes any direct input from patients—one of the main stakeholder groups whose privacy is at risk—or sometimes even from health care providers—another deeply affected stakeholder group. Patient preferences and utilities are represented only implicitly, and patients can voice their assessment of system design only indirectly by their decisions about where to go for care or by their pursuit of legal redress for damages resulting from lost privacy.

This chapter addresses the technological aspects of privacy and security in health care information systems. It outlines the types of technical security tools that can help manage security risks and then describes the types of tools used by health care organizations. It examines technological issues associated with patient identifiers and other means of linking patient records, and discusses the role of rights management technologies in imposing accountability and control on secondary uses of health information. Finally, the chapter examines obstacles that impede the more widespread use of advanced technical security practice in the health care industry.

---

[2]This statement does not minimize the difficulty of developing a quantitative metric of likelihood. Given the limited data available on violations of privacy and security, it is far more difficult to determine the likelihood of an insider leaking information than to estimate the likelihood of power outages based on good data obtained from the power company.

OBSERVED TECHNOLOGICAL PRACTICES
AT STUDIED SITES

Through its site visits and subsequent deliberations, the committee sought to determine what practices were currently in place in health care organizations, and whether these were prudent practices, as defined primarily in other non-health care settings. Most health care systems are very heterogeneous, meaning that excellent security practices may be in effect in some localized subsystem, but may be entirely missing in other parts of the organization (possibly violating the principle of balance). Thus, summary reporting on the security practices of a widely distributed organization is only a superficial approximation of the range of practices in force.

The committee examined a range of technological practices and mechanisms that can be organized into the following main areas:

- Authentication;
- Access control;
- Audit trails;
- Physical security of communications, computer, and display systems;
- Control of external communications links and access;
- Exercise of software discipline across the organization;
- System backup and disaster recovery procedures; and
- System self-assessment and maintenance of technological awareness.

These types of practices address different combinations of the five key functional areas of technological intervention listed above (Table 4.1). Authentication, for example, supports accountability, perimeter identification, access control, and comprehensibility. Physical security addresses system availability and perimeter identification. As a result, combinations of these practices are necessary for robust security.

These security considerations are focused on protecting information *within* provider institutions and do not address the problems of unrestricted exploitation of information (e.g., for data mining) after it has passed *outside* the provider institution to secondary payers or to other stakeholders in the health information services industry. A relatively new technological approach (rights management software) is discussed below in "Control of Secondary Users of Health Care Information" that may help in controlling the use of information both across and within organization boundaries.

The following sections discuss in more detail the eight categories of

TABLE 4.1 Functions Served by Different Technological Mechanisms

Mechanism	Function					
	Availability	Accountability	Perimeter Identification	Access Control	Comprehensibility and Control
Authentication		x	x	x	x
Access control		x	x	x	x
Audit trails		x		x	x
Physical security	x		x		
Control of links	x		x		
Software discipline	x	x	x	x	
Backup and disaster recovery	x				
System self-assessment	x	x	x	x	

security practice described above and the committee's findings based on its site visits. These findings are reported in terms of examples of observed current practice in health care computing environments. As the committee's site visits revealed, the protection of patient information could be greatly improved if existing, but currently undeployed, technologies were brought into more routine practice in health care settings. Specific technologies include strong cryptographic tools for authentication (Box 4.1), uniform methods for authorization and access control, network firewall tools, more aggressive software management procedures, and effective use of tools for monitoring system vulnerability. In the discussion below, instances in which other undeployed technologies could improve security are pointed out. Obstacles to the use of these tools and techniques are addressed later in the chapter.

Authentication

Authentication is any process of verifying the identity of an entity that is the source of a request or response for information in a computing environment. It is the linchpin for making decisions about appropriate access to health care information, just as it is for controlling legal and financial transactions. Generally, authentication is based on one or more of four criteria:

1. Something that you have (e.g., a lock key, a card, or a token of some sort);
2. Something that you know (e.g., your mother's maiden name, a password, or a personal ID number);
3. Something related to who you are (e.g., your signature, your fingerprint, your retinal or iris pattern, your voiceprint, or your DNA sequence); or
4. Something indicating where you are located (e.g., a terminal connected by hardwired line, a phone number used in a callback scheme, or a network address).

These, of course, all depend on user's integrity in not sharing the key, token, secret, or characteristic that purports to identify them. The classical method for authentication in computing environments is to assign each user a unique identifier (user or account name) and to associate a secret personal password with each such account. IDs and passwords can work reasonably well but are subject to a number of problems. For example, besides sharing their accounts with others, users may forget their password or they may pick passwords that can be guessed easily. Passwords may also be compromised if users write them down where others

BOX 4.1
Cryptographic Technologies

At present two kinds of cryptography are of potential use: symmetric or secret-key cryptography, a system in which the same key is used for encryption and decryption, and asymmetric or public-key cryptography, a system in which two different keys are used, one for encryption and one for decryption. The most common secret-key system in use today is the Data Encryption Standard (DES) developed by IBM and the National Bureau of Standards in the early 1970s and adopted as a federal standard in 1976.[1] DES uses a 56-bit key to encrypt and decrypt information based on a bit manipulation algorithm that is well suited to rapid execution on modern computers. Because only a single key is involved, it must be shared (and therefore transported) between parties wishing to exchange information securely. Safe key transport can be a major problem.

The most common public-key system available today is the Rivest, Shamir, Adleman (RSA) system patented in 1983. RSA depends on the difficulty of factoring very large numbers and uses Euclid's algorithm from algebra to define key pairs that are used to encrypt and decrypt information by modular exponentiation. The order of key use is commutative so that if data are encoded by key 1 of a set, key 2 is used to decode the data and if data are encoded by key 2, key 1 is used to decode them. Because two keys are required, only one need be kept secret by the user to whom the key set is assigned. The other (public) key can be made generally available. If the public key is used to encrypt information, the sender can be assured that only the holder of the (other) secret key can decrypt it. Similarly, if the holder of the secret key encrypts information, someone with the public key can be sure the information came from the secret key holder. With proper certification that a public key is assigned to a given individual, this is the basis of the digital signature and related services.

Public-key systems run about 1,000 times more slowly than DES systems and require keys about 10 times longer.[2] For this reason secret-key cryptography and public-key cryptography are often used together. Public-key cryptography is used for transactions in which the certified identity of the sender and/or receiver of a given message is crucial (and hence worth the computational cost). One such application is to transfer secure DES session keys to be used in higher-volume subsequent encrypted communication between entities.

---

[1] U.S. Department of Commerce, National Bureau of Standards. 1977. "Data Encryption Standard," *FIPS Publication 46*. National Bureau of Standards, Washington, D.C.

[2] Diffie, Whitfield. 1988. "The First Ten Years of Public-Key Cryptography," *Proceedings of the IEEE,* Vol. 76, No. 5, May, pp. 560-577.

SOURCE: Computer Science and Telecommunications Board, National Research Council. 1996. *Cryptography's Role in Securing the Information Society.* National Academy Press, Washington, D.C.

can see them or if they are sent across communication lines in an unencrypted form.

Log-in credentials (accounts, passwords, physical tokens, etc.) must be linked closely to the user's employment status or relationship to the organization. Often information is slow to propagate through the organization to individual system managers when the status of a user changes: students and temporary workers come and go and employees terminate or are terminated. Leaving system accounts accessible after a user no longer has rights of access is a major source of security vulnerability.

Authentication Technologies Observed on Site Visits

As might be expected with the rapidly evolving computing environments of today's health care organizations and the integration of many legacy information systems with more modern ones, there is little uniformity in the use of authentication methodologies. Many systems are dependent on the authentication procedures built in by the vendor, and the lengths and formats of valid account names and passwords are often incompatible.

The most common practice in the sites visited was the use of unique account IDs (generally assigned by a system administrator) and conventional unencrypted passwords for each individual user. Often some attempt was made to ensure that users chose difficult-to-guess passwords and that passwords were changed every few months, but enforcement was lax. In many environments, users must remember multiple passwords, depending on which information server they are accessing, and the trade-off is user convenience (not forgetting passwords) versus security. In situations with complex or rapidly changing passwords, users are often tempted to write down the codes for easy reference, most often in personal notebooks but sometimes on slips attached to their workstations, although the committee did not observe passwords written openly during its site visits. Where password changes are required periodically and the new password is not allowed to be the same as the previous one, the most common practice was to have two easy-to-remember passwords that the user alternated between at change intervals. Controls over passwords and account deactivation were most rigorous in centrally controlled systems and became much more relaxed in more decentralized and loosely affiliated groups.

The strongest practice observed was the experimental use of centrally issued user token cards (magnetic strip swipe cards) in conjunction with a user's personal identification number (PIN). This scheme was applied to only one of the clinical information systems in the organization, and the software to support it was written in-house. User acceptance was high and was enhanced by the fact that the swipe card served other uses such as parking lot or building entry authentication. Other examples of strong authentication technologies included localized use of encrypted password-checking schemes for modem dial-up services, although subsequent communications across the network were generally unencrypted. Such examples of good authentication technology usage were rare and were not deployed organization-wide across information resources.

One weak practice observed by the committee was the use of systems in a few sites where the user ID and authentication functions were combined into a single PIN. Each user had a different PIN, but the PIN was so short that a large fraction of all possible PINs was being used, and it was relatively easy for an unauthorized user to guess a usable PIN. An even weaker practice observed at one site was the use of common shared log-in accounts for large classes of providers with shared (and widely known) passwords—e.g., a common account password shared by all physicians and another by all nurses (passwords such as "doc"). Such systems provide almost no protection and depend entirely on the ethical integrity of the entire population of providers, administrators, patients, and visitors— a practice workable in only the most fortunate of organizations.

Some sites use a location-based authentication system. For health care systems, the committee believes that authentication based solely on the location of the user is very weak and should be used only under very exigent and carefully controlled circumstances. First of all, with the proliferation of personal computers and the use of high-speed packet-switched communications systems, many users move from machine to machine in the course of their workdays and there is no single applicable location. Second, network addresses change often enough to make it difficult to keep the location database up-to-date and validated. Third, it is relatively easy to fake (Internet) addresses in current communications systems so that apparent location is not a useful or verifiable criterion for identification. Location-based denial of access is used in some sites and may be a helpful adjunct to access control (see below), but it is not sufficient for authentication.

Authentication Technologies Not Yet Deployed in Health Care Settings

In addition to procedures that strengthen the use of passwords by requiring users to change them frequently, employing codes that are hard to guess, and instituting incentives or sanctions against sharing them, a number of technological schemes are available to strengthen the use of passwords. These are not in general use in the health care industry but include single-session passwords (those that are valid for one log-on session only), encryption technologies (either secret or public key), and "smart cards" (described below) or other tokens (e.g., the swipecard in limited use at one of the sites the committee visited). Each of these approaches helps avoid exposing passwords to snooping when the user's identity is being verified, and cryptographic tools provide stronger validation of the source and content of information sent between machines.

The most prudent and safe approach to authentication today in health care environments appears to be the use of a unique account identifier for each user with an encrypted password or PIN system (e.g., a secret or public-key Kerberos system as described below) in conjunction with a token. Both the password and the token must be presented to identify a user. This approach combines something you know with something you have and will be the basis, for example, for authentication in Internet commerce systems. Furthermore, this kind of password-token approach can be used for organization-wide identification so that users need be asked only once to log into the organization environment and thereafter have access privileges based on the role they fulfill and the information service they attempt to access, no matter where it is located in the organization.

Kerberos Organization Authentication. An important system for organization authentication of users, clients, and servers is called *Kerberos.* Kerberos was developed at the Massachusetts Institute of Technology (MIT) as part of Project Athena in the mid-1980s.[3] The central contribution of Kerberos is the practical management of secret keys for secure communications among thousands of workstations in a distributed organizational computing environment. The current Kerberos implementation functions without public-key encryption technology, yet limits the number of secret keys that must be used in an interconnected system. For example, in a simplistic system, if each of 1,000 users in an organization is to communicate securely with any of the other 999 workstations, the system must generate a unique password for each possible combination of workstations. This implies managing some 1,000,000 keys (1,000 possible senders times 1,000 possible recipients). If on the other hand a central key distribution service existed that could dispense secret keys securely to pairs of users as needed for communications, then on the order of 1,000 fixed keys would be needed—one for each user to employ in communi-

---

[3]See Miller, S., C. Neuman, J. Schiller, and J. Saltzer. 1987. "Section E.2.1: Kerberos Authentication and Authorization System," *MIT Project Athena,* Cambridge, Mass. See also Needham, R., and M. Schroeder, 1978, "Using Encryption for Authentication in Large Networks of Computers," *Communications of the ACM,* Vol. 21, No. 12; and Kohl, J., and C. Neuman, 1993, "The Kerberos Network Authentication Service (V5)," RFC 1510, Internet Working Group, available on-line at http://ds.internic.net/rfc/rfc1510.txt.

cating with the key distribution center (KDC). The Kerberos system takes such an approach and has to manage a number of keys that is directly proportional to the number of users in the organization. It distributes time-limited secret session keys without the need for passwords to pass in cleartext over any part of the computer network. Although the KDC represents a focal point of vulnerability in the system, Kerberos is a major step forward in organization management of secure communications and is the basis of strong authentication in the Distributed Computing Environment being promoted by the Open Software Foundation (OSF). Kerberos is being used actively in some health care and other facilities that the committee did not visit, in which secure authentication of more than 30,000 entities is required.

Smart Card Tokens. Internet commerce interests are pushing forward aggressively on standards for developing and deploying token-based cryptographic authentication and authorization systems (e.g., the Mastercard-Visa consortium and CyberCash Inc.). These technologies should be adapted to health care organization and interorganization applications, including the establishment of certification authorities with adequate trust levels to be effective in health care settings. Commercial deployment of these technologies will drive the prices of tokens and related software down to the point at which they can be used cost-effectively for protecting access to personal health care information, and user acceptance will be high because use of the technologies will be familiar in other settings. In support of this direction, health care organizations, elements of the health care information services industry, professional organizations, and government agencies should strongly support the development of Internet and commercial efforts in this arena.

One example of a smart card token is a card about the size of a credit card but somewhat thicker that has a liquid crystal display in which a number appears that changes every minute or so (the length of the number and frequency of change depend on the card model). Each user card generates a unique sequence of numbers over time, and, through a shared secret algorithm, servers for which the user has been assigned access privileges can generate the corresponding sequence of numbers. Since only the bona fide user (nominally) possesses the card and the number sequence is unique, the number at any given time is used as a session password. Any snooper who detects the number being sent over the network must replay it within the cycle time of the card; otherwise a new random number, known only to the holder of the card, is required for log-in. Other devices suitably packaged as buttons, smart cards, or similar tokens are becoming available at economically affordable prices. These have write-controlled internal memory (devices with 8 kilobytes of storage are readily available today) along with processing capacity to support services such as user-specific information storage, authentication, and cryptographic certificate management. Some even have biometric access control features.

Biometric Authentication Technologies. Various systems that measure the physical features of an individual (e.g., fingerprints, voiceprints, retinal or iris patterns of the eye, hand geometry patterns, or facial features) or the features of repetitive actions (e.g., signature dynamics) have been studied as the basis of identification systems.[4] Such biometric systems have the potential advantage of convenience and difficulty in forging an access pattern, since the basis of identification is always physically with the subject and is typically a complex pattern. However, biometric systems must be evaluated in terms of their reliability (false-positive and false-negative identification rates), the time and user frustration involved in the repeated authentication attempts that may be needed, and the difficulty of fooling the system with simulated patterns. The most extensive objective measurements of the reliability of biometric methods have been done by Sandia National Laboratories.[5] These studies evaluated a number of commercial systems using voiceprint analysis, signature dynamics, retinal patterns, iris patterns, fingerprint analysis, and hand geometry. The Sandia data indicate that the most effective technologies currently available for identification verification (i.e., verifying the claimed identity of an individual who has presented a magnetic stripe card, smart card, or PIN) are systems based on retinal or hand geometry patterns. These systems have one-try false-rejection and false-acceptance rates of less than 1 percent. User pattern collection and verification processing take about 5 to 7 seconds. Biometric systems have already progressed to the point at which they are being put into operation to help verify identities in applications such as personal and electronic banking, human and social services delivery, driver's license verification, industrial security, immigration control, and other settings where convenient, nonforgeable identification is necessary.[6]

---

[4]See, for example, Daugman, J.G. 1993. "High Confidence Visual Recognition of Persons by a Test of Statistical Independence," *IEEE Transactions on Pattern Analysis and Machine Intelligence* 15(11):1148-1161.

[5]Holmes, J.P., L.J. Wright, and R.L. Maxwell. 1991. "A Performance Evaluation of Biometric Identification Devices," Sandia Report SAND91-0276. Sandia National Laboratories, Albuquerque, N. Mex., June. See also Bouchier, F., J.S. Ahrens, and G. Wells. 1996. "Laboratory Evaluation of the IriScan Prototype Biometric Identifier," Sandia Report SAND96-1033. Sandia National Laboratories, Albuquerque, N. Mex., April.

[6]See, for example, *Biometrics in Human Services User Group Newsletter*, Vol. 1, No. 1, July 1996.

Access Controls

Once a user is identified, the next step is to determine the privileges that user has in terms of accessing services and information. This requires determining access both to particular application programs and to particular sets of data. In environments in which there is no notion of organization log-in, the existence of an account for a user is the first order of access control. In a more general distributed framework, either a database must exist that contains information for each user regarding access privileges or each piece of information must be tagged to describe its access rights. The classical approach in a hierarchical file structure is protection assigned at each node—directory or file. More fine-grained systems would assign protection levels to individual data elements within each directory or file. Protections are usually assigned to control ability to perform operations on the data structure, for example, to read, write, append, delete, and create. Each node typically has an owner and a set of privileges that apply to that person, a set of privileges that apply to specially defined groups of users, and privileges that apply to everyone else. In more modern systems, quite general access control list (ACL) mechanisms are available under which each group of users may have its own set of privileges and additional privileges can be defined (e.g., whether an entity may even see that a node exists in the file structure). Similar access control mechanisms are implemented in commercial database systems and may apply at various levels of granularity in the data structure—database, table, record, or data element.[7]

Operationally the problem becomes one of securely maintaining the database of user privileges, assigning group memberships (roles) appropriate to the user's current function, and assigning appropriate role-based access controls to various elements of information, based on need and right to know. This operational process, of course, has little to do with technology deployment, except insofar as technology may provide a smoothly integrated user interface for managing the database of access information in a consistent and timely way. The difficulties that confound this process include not having a clear model for information secu-

---

[7]Note, however, that organizing all data in concert with all possible access rights is a major effort. Such a task requires that the many pieces of information contained within an electronic medical record be reviewed to ensure that retrieval of a given piece of information is consistent with all relevant access rights. This task is complicated by a number of factors. For example, not all data within a given electronic medical record are necessarily controlled by a single system or system supplier. As important, it is difficult to ensure that all data are properly filed, so that a partitioned access right will not retrieve any data that give or allow inferences beyond the authorized access rights.

rity (i.e., what information should be assigned what access controls), having multiple access privilege databases in an organization that must work in consort, and keeping track of the users in an organization and their often changing roles over time (e.g., providers who move from service to service or fill in temporarily for a colleague).

An additional crucial aspect of data access control for health care settings is to allow access overrides in the case of an emergency. When a patient shows up in an emergency care facility unconscious or incoherent, the physician, who may never have seen the patient before, must have access to crucial information (prior history, current medications, allergies, possible psychiatric status, etc.) quickly to make possibly life saving decisions about care. Thus, the context (urgency) of the need to know may override conventional access control mechanisms (with an appropriate audit log of the event, as described below).

Access Control Technologies Observed on Site Visits

The committee's review indicated that most health care organizations are attempting to adapt access control criteria and processes from paper record systems to on-line systems. Thus, most sites conceptually identify four classes of information:

1.   Public information (e.g., promotional materials, educational materials) available to any interested person inside or outside the organization;

2.   Internal confidential information (e.g., organizational policies, business strategies, outcomes and utilization information) accessible on a need-to-know basis to organization employees and affiliates;

3.   Confidential patient record information—the routine content of patient health records—accessible on a need-to-know basis to providers and oversight groups, as well as to outside groups (e.g., insurance payers); and

4.   Highly sensitive patient record information (e.g., records of celebrities or other widely recognized persons, or special content such as information related to substance abuse, psychiatric care, physical abuse, HIV status, and abortions) accessible on a restricted need-to-know basis to authorized users of patient record information.

Although these distinctions are made in principle, often information is not labeled appropriately, except for patient records and sensitive information; in fact, most organizations have not yet decided whether or not to put highly sensitive information on-line because of concerns about patient privacy. For medical record information, most sites do not distin-

guish access privileges among providers. Physicians approved for practice at an organization generally have access to any record they claim to
need, without further review. At the paper record level, where records
must be checked out of storage areas, the decision is generally made on
the basis of the number of records requested. If a provider requests more
than about three records at a time, questions are raised as to the purpose
and authorization, with the implicit assumption that some research project
is involved for which prior approval of an institutional review board is
needed.

The committee found strong pressure from physicians at the sites
visited not to distinguish record access privileges among in-house physicians based on any role-specific criteria. Their arguments included their
already strong ethical training and commitment to maintaining patient
privacy. In the small number of sites where role-based access controls
were being instituted, strong pressures were felt in the workplace setting
to broaden the access privileges for each role category because of providers' experiences with blocked access to portions of records that they felt
they needed in the course of their work. Such difficulties might be overcome by allowing user-initiated overrides in exceptional cases, followed
by audit to ensure that a legitimate need for the override existed. For
example, an exceptional access might trigger an automatic e-mail notification to the physician of record and an entry noting the access placed in the
patient's chart. In secondary use areas, such as insurance payers, the
committee observed that such role-based access control was not questioned and was in more routine use.

Some sites allow broad access privileges for providers but make it
clear that an audit trail (see below) is being kept of each access and that
perceived inappropriate use will be questioned and follow-up sanctions
applied. Evidence indicates that this kind of audit approach is effective as
a deterrent for providers based on principles of ethics. No site questioned
the need for emergency override for access to records, with provision for
possible after-the-fact audit analysis. The committee found no evident
use of strong authorization controls based on access control lists.

Other sites use a system that limits the databases and applications
that can be accessed from particular locations. For example, workstations
in the payroll department cannot access clinical databases even if the user
has the appropriate (role-related) authorizations. Similarly, workstations
in clinical settings may not access personnel files. Such restrictions must
be viewed as a means of supplementing rather than supplanting access
controls based on strong user authentication and need-to-know criteria.
Location-based controls can help define the access perimeter of information systems by preventing any users lacking appropriate authorizations

from accessing a system from a location not reasonably associated with a need for that data.

Access Control Technologies Not Yet Deployed in Health Care Settings

Access Control List and Role Based Access. The committee believes that the flexibility of access control list technologies, such as those being deployed in the Open Software Foundation's Distributed Computing Environment, should be deployed more widely to facilitate detailed management of information access based on often changing user role(s), temporal variations in role, and so forth. Several research studies and demonstrations of role-based access control are under way that may help in defining ways to manage the complexities and promote the use of this type of authorization.[8]

Anonymous Patient IDs. The health care community typically assumes that a patient's name (and other personal demographic information) is routinely associated with all steps in the patient's care—for example, chart information, blood and tissue samples, laboratory tests, radiological films, pharmaceuticals. This practice constitutes implicit open visual access to aspects of patient information on the part of all persons involved in a patient's care, even if they have no need to know the identity of a patient. This in turn often leads to breaches of privacy through disclosure of private information about acquaintances. It may be possible to reduce these frequent, casual, and accidental disclosures of confidential information if unique identifiers, other than the patient's name, were used on records, orders, testing, and diagnostic procedures, except where absolutely essential. For example, there is not always a need to have a patient's name displayed in processing laboratory or pathology data, or in analyzing radiology or cardiology test results, in many other situations.[9] A coded patient ID would suffice in many cases, just as bank account numbers and credit card numbers provide the true identifying label for financial trans-

---

[8]See Ferraiolo, David, and Richard Kuhn, "Role-based Access Controls," a summary of ongoing work at the National Institute of Standards and Technology, available on-line at http://nemo.ncsl.nist.gov/rbac/; and Wiederhold, Gio, Michel Bilello, Vatsala Sarathy, and XioaLei Qian, 1996, "A Security Mediator for Health Care Information," *Proceedings of the 1996 AMIA Conference*, Washington, D.C., October, pp. 120-124.

[9]In some cases, the use of patient names for laboratory tests is helpful. As one reviewer noted, on evening and night shifts when staffing is short, hospital laboratory personnel (who themselves often must draw specimens from patients in their rooms) must informally prioritize sampling. The more anonymous the specimens, the less likely is this informal—but important—information exchange and judgment to be made.

actions. Even though some laboratories prefer to match name and ID number to ensure the proper flow of data to patient records or require signed consent forms to accompany a specimen (particularly for HIV tests), laboratory technicians have no real need to know the names of patients whose samples they are analyzing, as long as the correct result occurs (i.e., the data are bound without error or ambiguity to the proper record). Only at a few points in the overall health care process is it necessary that the patient's full identity be known. Using session identifiers in place of the full patient name is equivalent to using access tickets in the Kerberos system for distributed computing authentication and authorization control where actual user or client identity is not carried in the ticket and is available only by means of authorized requests to the key distribution center. Similar capabilities are being developed for Internet commerce, where user anonymity is desired in the context of authenticated transactions (e.g., digital voting, anonymous digital "cash" purchases, and anonymous e-mail for suggestion box submissions). Such a system would preserve patient anonymity more effectively, preventing inappropriate access to patient-identified information while allowing information to be associated accurately with the proper patient record.

Audit Trails

As discussed in Chapter 3, there are basically two kinds of interventions for minimizing violations of the confidentiality of health care information: (1) obstacles such as strong authentication and authorization technologies and (2) deterrents such as threats that misbehavior will be observed and sanctions applied. In a health care setting, obstacle-like remedies have limited effectiveness because they often cost time and aggravation for providers carrying out their necessary tasks. Deterrents can be highly effective among groups such as health care providers, who are ethically motivated, or among groups that can be influenced by sanctions such as job loss or legal process.

Audit trails, or records of information access events, can provide one of the strongest deterrents to abuse. Audit trails record details about information access, including the identity of the requester, the date and time of the request, the source and destination of the request, a descriptor of the information retrieved, and perhaps a reason for the access. The effectiveness of such a record depends on strong authentication of users having access to the system; it does little good to know that a celebrity's health care record was retrieved improperly if it is impossible to determine the identities of all those who actually retrieved the record. Audit trail information must also be kept in a safe place so that intruders cannot modify the trail to erase evidence of their access. Finally, although there is some benefit in users' *thinking* that an audit trail is being kept and analyzed, such trails are truly effective only if their information is *actually* reviewed and analyzed.

Audit Trail Technologies Observed on Site Visits

The committee's site visits revealed that almost all organizations keep audit trails for access to information in central health care information systems, but they do so only inconsistently for secondary information systems. Management at one site believed that audit records were being kept but was not sure and did not feel that this was a problem because the *belief* that audit records were kept was enough to deter inappropriate behavior. In almost all sites, audit records were not reviewed until a complaint was received from a patient or employee who had alleged a breach of confidentiality. Follow-up was then generally a manual process of reviewing audit records and investigating the details of possible indications of misuse. Many of the sites visited by committee members display warning messages about audit review to users accessing sensitive information.

Another site allows employees to review all accesses to their own medical records (most workers in health care organizations receive personal care in their employing organization). Employees can, at the touch of a button, generate a list of all users who accessed their record over a specified period of time. Most employees reported that they check their access logs regularly after receiving medical treatment and check them periodically in between treatments to detect any unusual accesses. Although such reviews only rarely detect unwarranted accesses, both management and staff report that the capability has heightened workers' appreciation of patients' privacy concerns and has helped educate them about the legitimate flows of health care data throughout the organization (to physicians, nurses, billing clerks, etc.). All see it as a successful deterrent against internal abuses of privileges.

Audit Trail Technologies Not Yet Deployed in Health Care Settings

There is wide agreement that audit trails deter unethical use of health information insofar as breaches can be detected and sanctions instituted against abusers. Currently audit trail analysis is almost entirely manual, and as a result, audit trails are rarely scanned unless a misuse is suspected based on external evidence. Only a few of the sites visited used any sort of automated audit trail analysis or exception-reporting programs. The site that had the capability to display audit logs routinely for its own employees had developed software tools to extract a single thread of patient-specific record accesses from the huge volume of audit trail entries.

Another site has a system that collects data prospectively on the legitimacy of access to records. For every access to data, the system displays a short checklist of reasons for access (e.g., providing care, quality review, billing, and so on). The checklist varies, depending on the requester's role, and is derived from context information such as patient-provider relationships, ward or bed assignments, and past access patterns. If the appropriate reason is not listed in the checklist, the requester types the reason in a text field. If the requester is a primary caregiver, access is assumed to be legitimate, and no reason is requested; any other provider who claims to be caring for the patient is approved for a six-month period of time. Quality review requesters are asked again after one week, on the assumption that their study should not require them to keep accessing a record for longer than that. Those looking at the record because they are merely trying to identify the right patient would be asked again on the next access. In most instances, the extra cost to the user is just to hit an OK response. In addition to these records being kept for possible future audit, all accesses are also reported to the patient's primary care provider, who can use this information to detect unwarranted snooping. When given the opportunity to turn off this reporting function, about half of the doctors chose to do so and not receive such notifications. This arrangement may provide an important basis for detecting suspicious accesses flagged by automated audit software and forwarded for human review.

More effective software tools are needed to maintain continuous surveillance of audit trail information so that abuses are detected quickly and sanctions meted out, both to maintain the effectiveness of audit trails as prevention tools and to contain, as soon as possible, the extent of any abuse. Such tools must be relatively sophisticated and take into account expected usage patterns and auxiliary information, such as appointment schedules and referral orders, in order to minimize the false-positive and false-negative rates in audit trail analyses. Criteria for access review might include claimed emergency need, any access to a celebrity record, access at a time or from a location out of the ordinary for a given provider, or access to a record by a provider for whom no recent appointment or referral record is available.

Physical Security of Communications, Computer, and Display Systems

Physical security entails appropriate controls to prevent unauthorized people from gaining access to an organization's information systems, including workstations, servers, and displays, so they cannot tamper with or derive information from the equipment. These controls can include such practices as positioning monitors and keyboards so they cannot be seen easily by anyone other than the user, or locating workstations that are used only intermittently (e.g., those in an examination room or an interview room near the main lobby) behind locked doors. Physical security is not a substitute for other security measures such as authentication and access control, but it can supplement these practices by limiting exposure of the information systems to unauthorized users.

The ability to implement strong physical security depends on knowledge of the inventory and configuration of communications and computing equipment in an organization so that appropriate controls can be implemented. For example, to manage internal network security properly, system managers must know the configuration, composition, and layout of network communications facilities within an organization so they can identify potential areas of vulnerability. These issues become especially important as the number of devices in a typical health care organization grows to tens of thousands and operational control over configurations, locations, connectivity, software census, and so forth becomes increasingly complex.

Physical security also requires that outdated computing equipment be disposed of properly.[10] Given that the average time to turn over computing equipment in the rapidly evolving marketplace is between 1.5 and 3 years, the proper disposal of equipment, media, and other materials that contain confidential information is essential. Sending a machine to an external contractor for repair with a disk that contains patient-specific information raises potential security problems. Deleting all files on a disk without degaussing or "wiping" the surface[11] leaves the contents of the disk intact for recovery by disk data structure analysis and reconstruction programs, potentially revealing confidential information previously stored on the disk. Similarly the disposal of backup tapes, floppy disks,

---

[10] In one instance, a commercial typing service that had been under contract to a local hospital went out of business. Its computer disks eventually were offered for sale at a local second-hand merchant—complete with patients' medical information that had never been erased. See Flaherty, David H. 1995. "Privacy and Data Protection in Health and Medical Information," notes for presentation to the 8th World Congress on Medical Informatics, Vancouver, B.C., Canada, July 27 (available on-line at latte.cafe.net/gvc/foi/presentations/health.html).

[11] Degaussing refers to a procedure in which the magnetically recorded ones and zeros that are the physical embodiment of data stored on a disk are erased. Wiping refers to a procedure in which random bits are written over the deleted data several times. Degaussing or wiping are not typically performed when a file is deleted by the operating system (this is the basis for "undelete" commands that recover deleted files).

and other media without degaussing can also lead to disclosure of confidential information.

The committee found that most of the sites visited had moderate physical security in place for their information systems; one site had somewhat stronger practices. The machines that provide centrally controlled services—mainframes and other production servers—were identified, located in very secure settings, and well controlled at the sites the committee visited. This derives from historical concerns in information systems departments for central equipment. In the strongest sites, support included excellent commercial-grade secure machine rooms with card-key access, alternative power, redundant storage for key file systems, and backup server equipment.

Outside the main server areas, however, physical security was much more relaxed. In organizations with 20,000 workstations of various sorts distributed throughout wide-reaching work locations, it is nearly impossible to maintain close physical control over the location of equipment and the means by which it is accessed. This does not mean there is no effort aimed at the physical security of these machines in the sites visited, just that the problem is operationally very difficult. Control of equipment in inpatient clinical care settings was tighter than in outpatient settings, and the least control was exerted over machines in research areas. Even in clinical settings, it was often difficult to control access to workstations and terminals so that the demands of work flow did not impede information security. For example, configuring terminals so that authorized clinical staff have easy access may conflict with a configuration in which unauthorized people are unable to look at display content, sit at an abandoned logged-in terminal, or snoop output at printers or paper disposal containers.

To prevent unauthorized users from gaining access to machines that are left unattended while logged on (and to prevent employees from working at such machines under another employee's ID), many of the sites visited programmed their workstations to automatically log-off or obscure screen contents after a specified period of time. Practices varied among locations within sites visited, depending on the set of applications accessible from a given workstation and the work flow within a particular setting. Computer terminals in nursing stations, for example, may typically wait longer before logging off than those in more accessible areas because nurses often need to walk away from terminals momentarily to check on patients or refer to other information. Workstations used by physicians for order entry may have to be programmed to log off more quickly, to prevent an unauthorized person from entering a false order. Some hospitals allow departments to adjust the log-off time within some specified parameters to fit in better with the needs of users. In several sites, log-in or screen-lock time-outs for unattended machines were eliminated or made very long for the convenience of busy clinical staff who did not want to bother with repeat authentication procedures.

Control of External Communication Links and Access

All of the sites the committee visited employ internal local area networks (LANs) to interconnect user client computers with information servers, and they often employ backbone links between multiple LANs within complex campuses or to connect LANs between geographically separate sites. Because physicians are mobile and need to access patient information from hospital and clinic sites and from home in off hours, external network or dial-up modem access is frequently provided as well. About half of the sites already have connections to the Internet, and those that do not are feeling pressures from providers and patients for Internet access.

Each type of external access to health care information resources poses possible security vulnerabilities that could compromise patient privacy. If a remote site uses weak authentication methods—enabling an intruder to easily pose as a trusted physician—and the remote network is connected directly to the information services of another site, the intruder can gain inappropriate access to confidential information. If a campus network is connected directly to the Internet (or to a widely distributed and open intranet), an intruder can install snooping software on an idle workstation and grab cleartext passwords or can exercise more sophisticated break-in scripts to exploit network service vulnerabilities and gain entry to confidential servers.

Although the committee's site visits did not reveal any substantial evidence of intrusions and misuse from this kind of external break-in, ample evidence at other commercial, academic, and government sites indicates that this threat is real and inevitable for health care organizations (see Chapter 3). Such unscrupulous intruders are often undeterred by ethical considerations or threats of audit trails; thus effective technical obstacles are necessary. The strong authentication and authorization technologies discussed above constitute a crucial element of prudent practice. Another important practice is to allow only few, well-defined, and very carefully monitored external access points to organization networks and information resources. One way to control external network access is to use firewall technologies.[12] A firewall is basically a single focused point

---

[12]Cheswick, William R., and Steven M. Bellovin. 1994. *Firewalls and Internet Security.* Addison-Wesley, Reading, Mass. See also Chapman, D. Brent, and Elizabeth D. Zwicky. 1995. *Building Internet Firewalls.* O'Reilly & Associates Inc., Sebastopol, Calif.

of entry for external users that can be configured and controlled to observe high security standards. This is done by requiring strong authentication and by allowing access only to trusted, essential services deemed necessary for organization business. Focusing access control efforts on a single firewall machine takes some of the burden away from having to fully secure many thousands of workstations otherwise accessible to outsiders. This is not to say that internal workstations should not be monitored and configured with secure software; rather, the firewall provides a more reliably effective first barrier to inappropriate entry.

A firewall normally sits between an internal trusted network and an external network connection either to the Internet or to an untrusted part of an intranet. In the most common configuration, a firewall consists of devices called a screening router and a bastion host. The screening router allows only messages from a specified list of trusted parties or locations to enter the system. Such requests are directed to the bastion host, which is configured securely to run only a limited set of trusted and necessary services for external users—for example, e-mail routing or remote terminal connections (with strong user authentication). Communication packets for authorized services are passed through "proxy" handlers in the firewall, which monitor packet types and sequences to give increased assurance of appropriate use. The router or firewall (1) should be configured to prevent users from making it appear as though they are trusted parties (in technical terms, it should prevent "spoofing") so that an outside workstation cannot appear to be an internal trusted workstation, (2) should prohibit unsafe connections (e.g., for the Network File Service protocol), (3) should prevent viewing internal Domain Name Service information (the host's Internet address information containing details about its internal network configuration), (4) should require direct console log-ins to control critical firewall system functions, and (5) should keep full audit trail information that cannot be modified once written.

Firewalls do not offer perfect protection; they are after all just another computer or software system. They may be vulnerable to so-called tunneling attacks, in which packets for a forbidden protocol are encapsulated inside packets for an authorized protocol, or to attacks involving internal collusion. Furthermore, firewalls check only the tags identifying various data packets, not the content of the packets being retrieved and, hence, depend on error-free organization of the domain they protect. Nevertheless they serve a useful purpose in focusing system administrator's attention on a smaller number of points of entry in a complex organization so as to control the most obvious kinds of attacks. Similar techniques can be used to control dial-up modem access to network services, again through the use of strong authentication techniques and limited service access.

Network Control Technologies Observed on Site Visits

Based on the committee's site visit review, all sites were acquainted with the threats from external access, and almost all of those sites with Internet connections used effective firewall technology to control unauthorized users. Expert attention was not always given to these issues though. One site claimed not to have an Internet connection but nevertheless was able to receive electronic mail from Internet sites. Sites without current Internet connection had plans to install a firewall along with any future connection. In those sites with extensive network connectivity, even if firewall technologies were used, limited effort was applied to monitoring break-in attempts, even though system administrators acknowledged that break-ins were feasible.

Connections from remote organization networks were much less carefully managed in that authenticated access to remote site networks was not ensured, yet once connected remotely, an intruder would have no problem connecting to any organization network or machine. Dial-up installations tended to use dated equipment and therefore provided little security protection against unauthorized use. One of the sites with quite up-to-date practices had a dial-in access system that uses commercially available cryptographic tools for user authentication; another site was experimenting with this technology. Some sites used a modem callback scheme, which offers improved security but may be subverted in some settings by not hanging up the line before callback. Also, in an era of portable laptop computers and increasingly mobile health care providers, it is very difficult to maintain callback lists adequately to allow bona fide access from needed sites. In the strongest sites, modem equipment was being upgraded to more modern and secure authentication technologies that do not depend on caller location, and old equipment normally was left inoperable unless specific arrangements were made for manual activation for a particular need (e.g., access by a remote service technician).

Network Control Technologies Not Yet Deployed in Health Care Settings

Firewall Technologies. More extensive use of firewall systems between geographically and administratively distinct sections of an organization intranet should become commonplace, along with more conscientious monitoring of firewall performance. Current firewall systems are often difficult to configure and maintain, however. Vendor refinement of these products should be strongly encouraged along with Internet and commercial research into improved tools to prevent and to detect misuse.

Wireless Communication Technologies. Only one site visited was experimenting with wireless communications for client computer access and had not put any service into routine use. That site fully recognized the security problems (e.g., interception of unencrypted transmissions) attendant on wireless systems. Another site is using satellite communication technologies to support telemedicine consultations and is taking the precautions of activating the links only during periods of operational use and of using encryption techniques to prevent unauthorized access. Wireless systems are expected to become much more commonplace in coming years, and adequate use of cryptographic tools, secure vendor products, and user-administrator education will be essential.

Independent Health Care Network. Just as firewall technology can help focus solutions to vulnerability concerns for organizational intranetworks in manageable interfaces, a national network dedicated to health care purposes would facilitate the security of health care information. The banking industry has developed an independent network over which most electronic financial transactions take place. Similarly, a number of government agencies concerned about security protection, such as the Department of Defense, Department of Energy, and National Aeronautics and Space Administration, also operate independent networks. To manage controlled access to health care information as time goes on, a dedicated health care network would focus interfaces with the Internet on controlled gateways and firewalls, offering a first line of protection under which individual health care organization networks could operate using additional access controls as appropriate. Because a network large enough to connect all players in the health care sector would connect a large part of the world, any such network also should be designed to use cryptographic and other information security technologies internally. The economics of such a network are clearly an important issue, but these may be mitigated because a dedicated network might merge naturally with communications systems being put in place for distributed organizational integration, telemedicine, and telecare.

Denial-of-Service Vulnerabilities. Computing systems are vulnerable to a variety of attacks that do not involve improper access to information content but deny access to services and information content to all users and hence render the system unusable for health care. Such denial-of-service attacks can be accidental or intentional and can take various forms, including disruption of environmental services (e.g., power, air conditioning, communications), exhaustion of system resources (e.g., memory, processes, file or swap disk space, access ports), or overloading of system services (e.g., high-speed pinging for network response, broadcast storms, setting up many partially opened connections, sending volumes of e-mail messages, fetching large numbers of Web pages). Protecting against such attacks is often difficult because they represent normal system usage carried to the extreme. Physical security of system resources and firewall protection for intranet access are both important steps, although the firewall itself is subject to service and resource overload attacks. Beyond that, system staff awareness and vigilance are essential, including the ability to identify the nature of a problem and trace the source to seek remedy. It is essential to keep up with community reports of vulnerabilities and solutions through agencies such as the CERT Coordination Center at Carnegie Mellon University.[13]

Encryption

Encryption technologies are the basis for many of the technological tools available to help secure computer-based information. Such technologies have received much attention in the popular press recently in terms of protecting Internet commerce, in terms of protecting the infrastructure of the Internet itself, and in terms of arguments for and against continued export control on products employing strong encryption tools.[14] Encryption can serve a number of uses in health care settings, including the following:

- Being the basis of strong user and computer authentication and access control;
- Protecting stored information or on-line communications against snooping or eavesdropping;
- Validating information content against unauthorized and undetected modification; and
- Validating the origin and content of physician orders, or other critical transactions and documenting the fact that they took place through the use of digital signatures.

Two points should be noted about cryptographic technology. The

---

[13]The CERT Coordination Center is the organization that grew from the computer emergency response team formed by the Defense Advanced Research Projects Agency in November 1988 in response to the needs indentified during the Internet worm incident. The CERT charter is to work with the Internet community to facilitate its response to computer security events involving Internet hosts, to take proactive steps to raise the community's awareness of computer security issues, and to conduct research targeted at improving the security of existing systems (see www.cert.org).

[14]Computer Science and Telecommunications Board, National Research Council. 1996. *Cryptography's Role in Securing the Information Society.* National Academy Press, Washington, D.C.

first point is that security tools based on cryptography are still largely undeployed *anywhere* in the public computing industry, much less in health care. In the sites visited, the committee found almost no use of encryption technologies except in a few localized experimental settings for authentication of users of clinical information systems and in one telemedicine link using special commercial equipment to protect video transmitted by satellite channel. Neither secret-key nor public-key encryption was in routine use as a basis for authentication, to protect information sent over the network against snooping, to protect the contents of on-line databases, to validate information content and transactions (e.g., digital time stamps, cryptographic checksums, digital signatures, and nonrepudiation of orders), or to encrypt backup media against off-line tampering or access. Although all sites were generally aware of the existence of encryption technologies, these were not yet seen as essential parts of the needed information system infrastructure.

Despite the ready availability of much cryptographic technology and numerous specifications for incorporating it into operational services, very few users of modern distributed computing systems actually take advantage of cryptographic protections. Perhaps the most common active uses are in secure telephone systems using the Secure Telephone Unit-III (STU-III) specification (mostly by U.S. government agencies) and the Lotus Notes messaging and collaboration system used within limited corporate enterprises. A number of universities have set up Kerberos-based authentication systems based on software exported by MIT; some groups are using Zimmerman's Pretty Good Privacy system to authenticate and protect e-mail traffic; and there is some use of a product called Secure Sockets to protect sensitive World Wide Web communications. However, these are isolated and represent a very small fraction of the overall user population and traffic on intranets or the Internet. Thus, the lack of vendor-supported products in this area may be seen as a major impediment to more routine use.

The second point is that cryptography does not solve the security problem—cryptography transforms the access problem into a key management problem. (In other words, the problem of protecting a large volume of unencrypted information in transformed into the usually easier problem of protecting a much smaller volume of information, specifically the keys needed for encryption and decryption.) Much of the current discussion about commerce systems, legally binding digital document management, and strong authentication centers on the problems of secure and certified key management. The foundation of strong, public-key-based user authentication is an infrastructure system by which unforgeable certificates are issued with public keys that are trusted and ensure that a key is associated with the stated person. This certificate authority acts much like a notary public in the signing of conventional legal documents, where the notary seal certifies that the document signature was performed at an indicated time and place by an identified person. The analogue to a notary in digital authentication is a "certification authority"—some third party that signs a certificate containing the user's identity and public key. In turn, the third party's key must be signed by a higher-level certification authority. This process of signing higher-level certificates continues until one reaches a trusted certificate known to everyone. Only a few examples of key management systems exist today, such as the military telephone communications system using STU-III, Lotus Notes, campus Kerberos deployments, and beginning experiments with public-key systems in Internet commerce (e.g., MasterCard-Visa). For Internet commerce, the banking system is stepping forward to attempt to provide this function. In a broader setting, it has been suggested that the federal government establish a certification authority system, perhaps administered by the U.S. Postal Service or the Social Security Administration, but these are only postulated mechanisms at this point. As the scope of key management services grows, trust in the integrity of key assignments tends to diminish, and the problems of revocation in the case of key compromise become much more difficult. However this key certification function is carried out, it is an essential part of the necessary infrastructure for public-key authentication and digital signature systems and for the economical development of commercially supported, trusted security tools based on these technologies. The technical community has only begun to demonstrate workable, trusted systems using modern cryptographic tools.

Software Discipline

Computer software is at the core of health care information system functionality—whether network communications tools, operating systems, database systems, user interface tools, back-office operations programs, administrative and clinical applications programs, word processing systems, electronic mail systems, World Wide Web (WWW) browsers, or information retrieval tools. The proper functioning and integrity of computer software used by the organization is one of the key pillars of maintaining health care information integrity, availability, and access control. Many of the pre-scripted attacks used by Internet intruders simply exploit bugs in operating system or network service software on various machines to gain unauthorized entry. Uncontrolled system software on machines in the organization may introduce viruses (programs that propagate themselves within distributed computing environments and can cause damage or interfere with operations); Trojan horses (programs that on the surface perform a legitimate function but which also or instead compromise confidential information such as passwords or provide special easy access paths for unauthorized persons); or programs that perform unauthorized functions in organizational environments (e.g., eavesdropping on cleartext network communications, interfering with network or system operations, copying displayed information to files or e-mail messages).

One of the most effective countermeasures is employee education. Most users are motivated by sound ethical principles but may not realize that when they bring a new program onto their machine from a friend or Internet site, the program may be contaminated with a virus or Trojan horse. Other ways of managing organizational software content include controlling the loading of unauthorized software by disabling floppy and CD-ROM drives on individual workstations; forcing workstations to obtain applications they run from organizational servers whose content is closely controlled; running software census programs that record versions, configurations, and cryptographic checksums of software loaded on distributed machines (e.g., using the program *tripwire*); scanning machines on the organizational network for unauthorized active service ports (e.g., using the SATAN script collection[15]); and prohibiting or logging all file transfers from outside the organization (e.g., through the file transfer protocol or WWW protocols). In general, it is dangerous to offer network services that are not needed and that do not perform an identified valuable function for organizational operations. Whenever a new service is enabled—for example, a new network service or some of the newer distributed software technologies such as Java and other component-based systems—testing should be extremely thorough and careful, and conducted in networking environments that are well monitored and isolated from the overall organization until confidence in proper function is established. New component-based software tools may both facilitate the more effective organizational management of distributed software and introduce new ways to bypass system administrator security controls. Adopt-

---

[15]SATAN stands for Security Administrator Tool for Analyzing Networks and is a testing and reporting tool that collects a variety of information about networked hosts by examining network services. It can report data, investigate potential security problems (with a simple rule-based system), and provide pointers to patches or workarounds. In addition to reporting vulnerabilities, SATAN gathers general network information (network topology, network services run, types of hardware and software being used on the network). SATAN has an exploratory mode that allows it to probe hosts that have not been explicitly specified; thus making it a potential tool for attackers. For more information see ftp://info.cert.org/pub/cert_advisories/CA-95%3A06.satan.

ing widely supported and tested standards wherever possible is to be desired.

Software Control Technologies Observed on Site Visits

As in other areas, with the rapidly evolving computing environments of today's health care organizations and the integration of many modern and legacy information systems, there is little uniformity in the control of software systems, and few vendor tools exist to help with this problem. Controls over system software were most rigorous in closed, centrally managed mainframe and server systems and became much more relaxed in more decentralized and loosely affiliated groups. In some sites visited, the committee observed that local workstation floppy drives had been disabled to prevent unauthorized software loading. In general, this was done incompletely, however, and in one site the administrators claimed that drives had been disabled but site visitors were able to mount a floppy disk on a machine in a public area. Another of the sites regularly runs a network software census program to keep track of what software (by name at least) is running on each workstation in the organization. None of the sites visited audited installed software to determine if unauthorized changes had occurred. Also, whereas most sites have experienced problems in the past with imported software viruses, no site regularly runs antivirus software across systems to prevent problems. Rather, antivirus software is used after the fact to clean up virus problems once they are detected. Most sites are wary of the general use of Web-related tools because these make software loading from network sites a matter of clicking a mouse button. In those sites running Web software with Internet connectivity, none has disabled downloading external files by internal personnel; they depend entirely on employee ethics, knowledge, and good judgment to protect software resources.

The weakest practices observed by the committee included essentially uncontrolled software content for workstations, especially in open research areas. At least one incident has been reported in which a student intern loaded break-in scripts onto an internal workstation and experimented with them (causing no apparent damage), but no routine software census procedures have been put in place even after this incident.

Software Control Technologies Not Yet Deployed in Health Care Settings

Industrial, academic, and government organizations all face major problems in managing software systems across distributed computing environments. For the longer term, the committee recommends strong support for the development of standards and the deployment of vendor-supplied tools for organizational integration of secure distributed computing. Candidates for infrastructure elements of such a suite of tools include OSF's Distributed Computing Environment (DCE), the Object Management Group's Common Object Request Broker Architecture (CORBA), secure World Wide Web access management tools, and the Java component-based Web browser extension technology. Desirable capabilities should include uniform client-server authentication tools, access control lists for authorization, encryption of all data messages, and use of digital signature and content validation tools so that trusted software can be used within reliably secure networked domains.

System Backup and Disaster Recovery Procedures

Despite the increased reliability of modern computing systems using technologies such as high-density integrated circuits, improved packaging techniques, and high-capacity storage media, operational systems do fail. Processors, memory, and disks sometimes fail; software occasionally runs amok; environmental failures such as power outages, floods, and earthquakes regularly occur; and users sometimes delete important files accidentally. To guard against these outages and losses, alternative power sources and processing facilities must be provided for the most critical systems, and up-to-date system file backups must be performed and media kept secure. Good practices to cover for these kinds of failures have been in place for decades, and lower-cost systems and peripheral equipment have made redundancy and backup more convenient and effective than ever.

System Backup Procedures Observed on Site Visits

In its site visits, the committee found excellent practices generally in place for centrally managed mainframe and server systems. At the strongest sites, an inventory of critical systems was in place along with an evaluation of the maximum outage that can be sustained for various information resources without affecting health care. This evaluation is used as the basis for guiding the purchase of redundant processing facilities and their location within campus sites unlikely to be affected simultaneously by any but the most disastrous environmental failures. Full system backups are done regularly and the content is stored at multiple sites to protect against destruction of a single focused site. Routine drills are run to practice switching from hypothetically damaged operational facilities to backup facilities and to restore damaged information in the event of peripheral storage failure. The strongest sites also have redundant network communications facilities in place, routed independently so that environmental or mechanical accidents (e.g., backhoe damage during construction) do not interrupt vital links beyond tolerable periods.

Backup procedures, redundant facilities, and practice drills are much less common in more decentralized and loosely affiliated equipment sites. Often, personal workstations are dependent on users themselves for regular backup, a procedure frequently forgotten in the press of routine work activities. As indicated above, almost no attention is paid in current operations to protecting the content of backup media against snooping, other than physical security in the strongest sites: intruders would have to enter a physically locked facility to steal tape copies of backup information. There is no use of encryption technologies or cryptographic checksum technologies to protect backup stores against snooping or theft or to detect points at which unauthorized modifications might have been made to software or other file system content.

System Backup Procedures Not Yet Deployed in Health Care Settings

One of the key future technological challenges comes from needing to back up increasingly large file systems; often these contain terabytes of information (1 terabyte = 10^{12} bytes) when radiological image data are stored on-line. Off-line or mirrored storage is still relatively expensive, and the long time required to fully back up such large file stores means that times between full dumps increase. Systems that use time-stamped incremental backups will have to become routine.

System Self-Assessment and Attention to Technological Awareness

Concerns about computer security have been voiced for decades—historically most loudly in areas of national security and business—and procedural and technological solutions have been worked out for all but the most assiduous kinds of attacks. More recently, with the growth of the Internet and distributed computing, these issues have been felt more broadly, and a whole new class of problems centered on powerful new means of remote access to computers of all kinds has raised additional security challenges. Again procedural and technological solutions have been devised that offer prudent protection but recognize that concerted, directed, professional attacks on almost any computer facility will likely succeed despite the most rigorous protection. However, these "prudent practice" solutions have not been adopted uniformly, partly because the number of affected computers has grown exponentially and partly because people responsible for these systems are not trained to select and apply these solutions or are unable to enforce workable solutions within an organization.

In 1988, the Defense Advanced Research Projects Agency began funding a computer emergency response team (CERT Coordination Center) at Carnegie Mellon University as a national resource for collecting information about Internet security problems and disseminating solutions. However, this dissemination process has been slow and spotty; for example, a recent CERT summary alert (CERT Summary CS-96.02) lists seven general areas of vulnerability:

1. Compromised system administrator privileges on systems that are unpatched or running old OS versions;
2. Compromised user-level accounts that are used to gain further access;
3. Packet sniffers and Trojan horse programs;
4. Spoofing attacks, in which attackers alter the address from which their messages seem to originate;
5. Software piracy;
6. Send-mail attacks; and
7. Network File System and Network Information System attacks and automated tools to scan for vulnerabilities.[16]

The existence of many of these problems and solutions for them were known as long as 3 to 4 years ago, yet systems are still in operation that do not employ the necessary safeguards. Much has been written in other forums about procedures for managing systems safely in modern networked environments.[17]

---

[16]Network File System, or NFS, is an Internet protocol (defined in RFC 1094; available online at http://ds.internic.net/rfc/rfc1094.txt) for remote access to shared file systems across networks. Several vulnerabilities exist in the NFS protocol that allow intruders to gain privileged system access, unless the ports used by NFS are protected by a firewall and other techniques, and care is taken to share file structures only among trusted hosts. Network Information Service, or NIS, is used among Sun computer systems for the administration of network-wide databases. A vulnerability exists in early versions of NIS that allows unauthorized users to obtain a copy of the NIS maps from a system running NIS. The remote user can attempt to guess passwords for the system using NIS password map information that might be obtained in this way.

[17]See, for example, Holbrook, P., and J. Reynolds (eds.), 1991, "Site Security Handbook," IETF RFC 1244, July; a draft revision dated June 1996 is under review (see http://www.ietf.org/html.charters/ssh-charter.html). See also Garfinkel, Simson, and Gene Spafford, 1996, *Practical UNIX and Internet Security*, 2nd edition, O'Reilly and Associates Inc., Cambridge, Mass.; Cheswick, William R., and Steven M. Bellovin, 1994, *Firewalls and Internet Security*, Addison-Wesley, Reading, Mass.; Khanna, Raman (ed.), 1993, *Distributed Computing: Implementation and Management Strategies*, Prentice-Hall, Englewood Cliffs, N.J.; and Neumann, Peter, 1995, *Computer Related Risks*, Addison-Wesley, Reading, Mass.

Although only limited network intrusions have been detected to date in the health care settings visited by committee members, this occurrence is very common in other settings—commercial, academic, and government. Because health care organizations are moving rapidly toward network-based distributed computing systems (as stated above, one organization already has more than 20,000 workstations in its network system), the committee believes strongly that it is prudent for health care settings to adopt good practice in evaluating system threats and vulnerabilities. Steps that should be taken include aggressively staying current with standards and technologies for security management and with the vulnerability experiences reported by other sites (e.g., through the CERT Coordination Center registry). A health organization-focused CERT-like group would provide a focal point for collecting and coordinating the dissemination of information about security problems and solutions. Such a forum would also serve to educate and share experiences among managers, administrators, and technical personnel and even to promote the establishment of standards for technology and procedures across health care organizations.

Sites should continuously appraise their system architectures, hardware and software technologies, and procedures to eliminate outdated components and practices in favor of more effective solutions. Sites should regularly exploit the same tools that intruders use to probe vulnerabilities in their systems, including network service script sets such as SATAN and password-cracking programs, and they should routinely use software protection tools such as virus detection software and software checksum protection (e.g., *tripwire*).

System administrators at most of the sites visited by the committee were broadly aware of these practices but, except for one site, did not have them in place in any operational sense. System groups tended to react in response to perceived or detected problems rather than to maintain proactive vigilance. Sites with the weakest practices simply discounted this class of threats or placed it at such low priority that no financial or staff resources were allocated to deal with it. It is unlikely that such sites would even know if intrusions into their systems had occurred.

SITE VISIT SUMMARY

Table 4.2 summarizes the various security tools, operations, and procedures the committee observed at the six health care sites visited. A check mark indicates that the security feature is actively supported at that site with state-of-the-art technologies and operational practice in such a way that the site could serve as an example for others to follow. Absence

TABLE 4.2 Summary of Security Tools and Practices Observed During Site Visits

Security Feature	Site					
	A	B	C	D	E	F
Authentication						
Individual user IDs and passwords	✓	✓	✓			✓
Token-based authentication (e.g., token plus password)						
Change passwords often						
No unencrypted passwords						
Uniform user IDs across organization		✓	✓			
Incentives to reduce key sharing	✓	✓	✓		✓	
Access Control						
Need to know, right to know			✓			
Access control list technology and management						
Role-based access profiles			✓			
Access overrides for emergencies						
Audit Trails						
Audit trails and self-audit					✓	
Software-based audit analysis						
Physical Security						
Terminal security						
Security perimeter, network layout			✓			✓
Network physical security			✓			
Server physical security	✓		✓	✓	✓	✓
Secure destruction of obsolete data or equipment						
Control of Links						
Firewall	✓		✓	✓		✓
Dial-in protections	✓					

continued on next page

TABLE 4.2 Continued

	Site					
Security Feature	**A**	**B**	**C**	**D**	**E**	**F**
Mobile access protection						
Intruder script protection						✓
Control Internet Protocol addresses			✓			
Encryption						
Cryptography-based authentication						
Encrypt network traffic						
Encrypt database contents						
Digital signatures						
Document integrity						
Transaction nonrepudiation						
Encrypt backup media						
Software Discipline						
Use antivirus technology			✓			
Checksum, validate software			✓			
Control user software						
Control PC software loading						
Network software census			✓			
Integrated software tools						
Backup and Disaster Recovery						
Backups, multiple storage sites	✓		✓	✓	✓	✓
Data content integrity						
Operations recoverability	✓		✓	✓	✓	✓
System Self-Assessment Evaluation, Staying Technically Current						
Run anti-intrusion programs			✓			
Vulnerability evaluation			✓			
Stay up on CERT alerts			✓			
Avoid or update obsolete technologies				✓		

of a check mark means that the site pays only minimal attention to the given security feature or, in the opinion of the site visit team, could have made significantly more effective use of existing, proven technologies and practices. These judgments may differ from those of individual site managers and system administrators, who judge the need for a particular precaution on the basis of the perceived threat (or lack of it) within the organization. These security considerations are focused on preserving information confidentiality within provider organizations and do not address the problems of unrestricted use of information (e.g., for data mining) after it has passed, with consent, outside the provider organization to secondary payers or to other stakeholders in the health information services industry.

KEY ISSUES IN USING TECHNOLOGY TO PROTECT HEALTH INFORMATION

In addition to securing health information systems, as described above, technical tools can play a role in protecting patient privacy by facilitating or impeding the distribution of health information. While advanced computing and communications technology, in general, facilitates the dissemination of health information, technologies exist that can help limit unauthorized or inappropriate distribution of health information. Such technologies include patient identifiers and other approaches for linking records contained in disparate databases, as well as rights management technologies for limiting secondary distribution of health information.

Patient Identifiers and Techniques for Linking Records

Developing robust methods of indexing and linking patient records is critical to ensuring that providers have reliable data on which to base medical decisions.[18] Patient-specific health care information must be bound uniquely and unambiguously to the person to whom it relates through the use of an identifying label such as a medical record number. To ensure that the identifier is unique, organizations must prevent assignment of the same number to two different patients; to ensure that it is unambiguous, organizations must prevent indexing of any single patient's

---

[18]Within the computer science community, data integrity and availability are considered an integral element of system security. See Computer Science and Telecommunications Board, National Research Council. 1991. *Computers at Risk: Safe Computing in the Information Age.* National Academy Press, Washington, D.C.

records by two or more different numbers. Otherwise it may be difficult to find all the data associated with a person.

In a traditional health care environment, each organization—whether a hospital, a physician's office, or a pharmacy—generates its own identifier for each new patient. That identifier is used for all transactions involving the patient and provider, but the identifier is different for each organization. Names and addresses are generally inadequate as unique identifiers because they are not necessarily unique within large populations of patients. As a result, health care organizations have developed other mechanisms for generating patient identifiers. Some assign patient numbers sequentially; as new patients register with the hospital, physican, or insurer, they are assigned the next number in sequence. Other organizations use the Social Security number (SSN), relying on the Social Security Administration to ensure that numbers are assigned uniquely and unambiguously.[19] Still others have their own specific algorithms for generating numbers. One site visited for this study generated identifiers from the patient's first and last names, year of birth, and gender using an algorithm developed for generating driver's license numbers. An extra "tie breaker" digit is used to differentiate between multiple patients with otherwise identical numbers.

Administering patient identifier systems can be a cumbersome task, especially in organizations with large patient populations. Patients change addresses frequently or report their names differently (using a nickname versus a full name or a maiden name instead of a married name); this makes it difficult to use demographic information to determine whether two records with different numbers actually belong to the same patient. As health care systems merge into larger enterprises and integrated delivery systems, they increasingly face the problem of integrating and linking records from organizations that used incompatible identifier systems. Each of the sites the committee visited is concerned with the problem of managing unique and consistent patient identifiers within its enterprise.

One proposal for addressing this difficulty is to assign each patient a universal identifier to be used throughout the health care system. The Health Insurance Portability and Accountability Act of 1996 (Public Law 104-191) directs the Secretary of Health and Human Services to promulgate standards for a universal health identifier by February 1998. The proposed identifier would be assigned to each patient, employer, health

---

[19]Not all Social Security numbers are unique or assigned unambiguously. There are an estimated 4 million to 12 million false, invalid, or ambiguously assigned numbers in the current system, although improvements in management of the SSN continue to reduce the rate of error.

plan, and health care provider in the United States. One candidate for the universal health identifier is the Social Security number. Use of the SSN appears to have many potential advantages: it is already the basis for the medical record number in many organizations (including Medicare) or is elsewhere contained in the medical record, and a system already exists for assigning numbers. Use of the SSN as a universal patient identifier, however, raises the concern that it might facilitate linking of medical records with other types of records that are also referenced by SSN, such as Social Security, employment, financial, and driving records.

To circumvent this problem, it may be possible to use a system in which individuals have different unique identifiers to index information about them in different domains such as health care, banking, and insurance. Thus, Social Security records could continue to be indexed by SSN, but driving records would use a different numeric scheme, as would medical records, educational history, and so forth. Someone who desires to collate these disparate data sets would find that they contain no convenient shared identifier. Collation would depend on the presence of other distinguishing data in each database, perhaps including name, address, and birthdate. Because each database is likely to contain different subsets of such data and because none of them alone is enough to identify someone uniquely, the collation process would be fraught with greater uncertainties, and would be more difficult and costly. Linking information between domains would require an overt act to translate different identifiers; however, those organizations with legitimate needs to link data could routinely collect the data necessary to create the links without requiring a universal identifier, though possibly at greater expense.

Cryptographic methods allow many other variations in identification schemes. The British Medical Association, for example, is encouraging adoption of an identifier scheme wherein the patient's identifier at any institution is computed from public information about the individual (name, part of the postal code, and date of birth) combined with a secret identifier unique to the institution.[20] Other options include the use of temporary pseudonymous identifiers for tracking independent pieces of data such as laboratory results.

Many managed care organizations and integrated delivery systems are addressing the records-linking problem by developing master patient indexes. Such systems allow records at each affiliated institution to retain their original identifiers, but generate an overall index listing the various

---

[20]See Anderson, Ross J. 1996. "An Update on the BMA Security Policy," *Notes of the Workshop on Personal Information Security, Engineering and Ethics,* University of Cambridge, England, June 21-22.

numbers by which each patient's records are referenced in different institutions. Several companies now offer a service for creating master patient indexes for health care organizations. Typically, they use demographic data and incident information to link patient records across the enterprise and can determine unambiguously the patient to whom all but a small percentage of existing patient records refer.

Another approach to linking records across disparate organizations is to rely not on a particular number but on a limited set of specific patient attributes. One experimental system that is taking this approach allows providers in the emergency rooms of three Boston area hospitals to query each other's clinical databases for information about patients.[21] Because the three hospitals have their own patient identifier systems, the experimental system uses four attributes to search for related records: first name, last name, date of birth, and gender. Each system returns only unambiguous matches to the requester. In its present form, this system may not be feasible for linking larger numbers of records over a larger number of organizations, but it does highlight the possibility that additional research may yield innovative ways of linking records that do not rely on a single, universal identifier (See Chapter 6, Recommendation 5).

Control of Secondary Users of Health Care Information

From a technical perspective, the problem of controlling the use of information among secondary users is analogous to the problem of controlling intellectual property rights for vendors of on-line publications and other valuable information. Instead of wanting to ensure payment for information access, however, health care organizations want to authenticate, authorize, and record who accessed what information and for what reason in the health care setting. One approach to this type of control may be to pursue adaptations of rights management technologies being developed to manage intellectual property rights.[22] Such software controls would operate internally within provider organizations and also externally, as records pass to payers and other secondary users. The essential elements of a rights control system include the following:

- Chunks of information (components of the patient record, includ-

---

[21]Kohane, Isaac S., F.J. van Wingerde, James C. Fackler, Christopher Cimino, Peter Kilbridge, Shawn Murphy, Henry Chueh, David Rind, Charles Safran, Octo Barnett, and Peter Szolovits. 1996. "Sharing Electronic Medical Records Across Multiple Heterogeneous and Competing Institutions," available on-line at www.emrs.org/publications/.

[22]See, for example, a description of IBM cryptolope technology: Rodriguez, Karen. 1996. "Pushing the Envelope," *Communications Week*, May 13, p. 37. Similar technology is being developed by Xerox and AT&T.

ing text, laboratory results, and images) to be transmitted outside the organization are encrypted by a server within a health care provider's information system. The encryption is designed so that the information can be accessed only by special software (possibly a Java "applet") with an encryption key supplied by the server on receipt of properly authenticated user credentials.

• Potential users authenticate themselves through one of the public-key schemes and present authorization credentials for access to an appropriate part of the record. Types of access might include viewing demographic information only; viewing details of the most recent provider visit; viewing the full patient record except for potentially sensitive areas; or viewing, printing, and copying the entire record. Each access request would be logged to ensure accountability, and the software would destroy the access key after each use so that subsequent uses require reauthentication.

• The user downloads special access software from the provider (or trusted third party) that contains a key to decrypt the document upon authentication and tracks the use of portions of the document according to authorized privileges. Viewing software must be secure against tampering, and the system must make it difficult to implement work-arounds, such as "screen scraping" and core dump analyses, that would give users uncontrolled access to the decrypted material. Some workers in this field have gone so far as to propose that this approach could succeed only in the context of closed "network appliance" machines to which the user would have no access for software reconfiguration. If the encrypted document were sent to other users, they could access it only with the viewer application supplied by the provider, which would require new authentication and authorization before allowing access.

Although it is unlikely that such a rights management system can be made foolproof against the most technically competent unethical user, it may provide an audit trail of access up to a point of abuse, including recording that a local copy has been made (presumably against privacy protection laws) or that an overt act to circumvent software controls had occurred. Further it might be possible cryptographically to watermark digital medical record documents with the identities of the users to whom they were issued in confidence so that if a subsequent inappropriate disclosure is made, its source could be identified.

An obvious extension of these ideas would be to use rights management inside organizations as well, to enforce organizational policy on data collection, access, and dissemination. For example, an organization could use rights management tools to ensure that clinical data cannot be collected or aggregated even by internal staff except with the approval of an institutional review board. Rights management tools, coupled with legal reform to define acceptable use and disclosure, may also make it feasible to deploy a uniform health care identifier system with appropriate accountability for bona fide use within the health care industry.

OBSTACLES TO USE OF SECURITY TECHNOLOGY

The move to computerized patient records is made more urgent by many pressures: the need to allow simultaneous access to records by various providers involved in patient care in modern streamlined clinical settings; the push toward increased cost-effectiveness, meeting the needs of highly mobile patients, regional integration of providers and referral systems, and the use of telemedicine and telecare; the push toward evidence-based care; the need to analyze outcomes and utilization; the need for better clinical research support; attempts to improve health through more thorough immunization and nutrition programs; and so on. Despite an aggressive move toward computerized health care records in recent years and ongoing parallel technological improvements, there are still many obstacles and impediments to achieving usable and secure systems. The following are the principal hurdles related to the use of security technology that the committee found.

Difficulty of Building Useful Electronic Medical Records

The challenge of developing digital health care record systems that are useful, efficient, and cost-effective has proved to be so difficult that deployment of *any* system that works in the clinical care arena is the primary priority. Security is often relegated a much lower priority in this process. One of the goals of computerized patient record systems is to make care more cost-effective while maintaining high quality. Although minimizing inappropriate, expensive tests and treatments is an important part of these goals, the most direct goal is to save provider time (i.e., allow providers to care for more patients in less time). To date, the committee has been unable to document any clinical information system that saves provider time overall. Stronger security measures can only exacerbate this shortcoming by creating more hurdles that a provider must overcome to use a system; thus, security is often sacrificed in the interest of user acceptance and efficiency. As one chief information officer of a large health care organization told the committee, "Every minute of time a system costs a user to enforce security controls is multiplied 20,000 times across our physician population, and this translates into the loss of real dollars." The transition period between paper-based records and electronic records adds to the cost and increases the threshold to move toward electronic medical records since health care organizations must manage both the old paper and the new electronic record systems at the same time.

Lack of Market Demand for Security Technology

Few organizations can afford to develop and integrate strong information security technologies into their operational systems. Until vendors incorporate stronger, integrated, standard, open technologies, reliance on old and vulnerable technologies for user authentication, access control, network protection, and so forth, will persist. This seems to be a chicken-and-egg problem, however. Although some vendors do not appear to put much effort into security mechanisms, others reported that they have invested considerable effort in developing sound security features in clinical information systems they were marketing, but that these features do little to enhance sales. Vendors contend that there is little market demand for security that can help motivate a vendor to invest heavily in it. If this is true, at least some vendors may be prepared to deliver stronger security capabilities quickly if health care organizations make those capabilities a requirement for future system purchases. This suggests that a two-pronged approach is needed: (1) make technological interventions more acceptable by making them less of an annoyance to users; and (2) increase purchaser awareness regarding security issues, thus creating a market demand for these technologies so that vendors will integrate strong security tools in health care information system products.

Organizational Systems Accumulate—They Are Not Designed

Many of the provider sites visited by committee members are in acquisition mode; that is, they are actively pursuing mergers and acquisitions of other health care providers with the hope of achieving economies of scale in managing a larger organization, benefiting from referrals of patients from larger and larger population areas, and reducing competition. The merger of diverse hospitals and clinics entails inheriting legacy information systems that do not communicate information well with each other, much less share a common security framework. Such systems are not designed but evolve within the exigencies of business goals. Relying on the overriding ethical behavior of providers within the systems, security integration and reinforcement often receive lower priority. At a technological level, it would help greatly if commercial tools were available to integrate legacy systems into modern distributed computing environments. Beyond that, however, many other database content inconsistencies have to be overcome, including patient identifier systems, database terminology, information types, and units of measurement.

Cryptography-based Tools Are Still Out of Reach

As noted in the discussion of encryption, there is almost no common use of cryptographic tools in any modern public distributed computing setting today. It seems clear that cryptography-based technologies and standards specification are available for inclusion in health care systems, but this has not happened to any real extent, except in a few specialized commercial products and in more adventuresome academic settings. Much more aggressive demonstration of these tools and their integration into real systems are needed.

Effective Public-key Management Infrastructures Are Essential but Still Nonexistent

The basis for many of the features desired for security in health care information systems depends on deploying public-key cryptographic technologies—authentication, digital signatures, information integrity management, session key exchange, rights management, and so on. Trusted and effective key management is at the heart of these tools but is not a well-established process at this time. Substantial challenges remain to demonstrate a key management system (or systems) that connects keys reliably with bona fide organizations, providers, patients, and service personnel; that provides rapid and unassailable operational verification of credentials; that makes theft of key information difficult in systems deployed to non-computer expert user groups; that enables recovery of information in the case of lost keys; and that ensures rapid revocation of compromised keys and prevents exploitation of compromised information with protection based on those keys. Preliminary efforts to establish public-key management infrastructures are under way in the banking and Internet commerce communities but, to date, nowhere in the health care industry. Such systems must be set up to certify provider organizations, physicians, nurses, and other support personnel, as well as patients themselves, and these must operate effectively, conveniently, and in a setting of unquestioned trust and confident risk management. Considerable challenges remain to demonstrate a key management capability that is usable for health care, and demonstration projects should begin at once.

Helpful Technologies Are Hard to Buy and Use

Providers can rarely afford to develop their own information systems, and those sold by most vendors do not offer organizational solutions for security controls. Thus, with the push to more distributed systems, providers are forced to put up with multiple, incompatible authentication and authorization technologies or to construct special solutions for parts of their organizations. The tools to manage heterogeneous computing environments in terms of security, reliability, and so forth are not well developed. Standard ways are needed to link component systems together that meet requirements and do not overburden the system administrator. A great deal of technology already exists that can help protect health care information, but much of it has not been brought into routine practice yet. Specific technologies include strong cryptographic tools for authentication, uniform methods for authentication and access control, network firewall tools, more aggressive software management procedures, and effective use of system vulnerability monitoring tools. Some of these technologies—token authentication cards, for example—have been relatively expensive for wide deployment in large organizations. However, the costs of these technologies are decreasing (through volume adoption and competition) at the same time that their usability is improving. The tools to manage software across distributed heterogeneous systems consisting of many thousands of machines and users, including program census management, version control, and integrity control, are poorly developed. Overall the lack of standards for security controls and for vendor products that interoperate between disparate systems means that chief information officers postpone decisions about implementing and enforcing effective security solutions.

Education and Demystifying Issues of Distributed Computing and Security

The revolution in distributed computing and communications systems that has been brewing since the 1960s and 1970s has taken hold full force in commercial organizations during the past decade. Health care organizations have been among the slowest to adopt these new technologies, however, and existing management and information systems personnel are not fully prepared. The lack of technical understanding, the lack of direct experience with these new tools, the lack of confidence in their management, the lack of a peer group of successful adopters (except for a few academic medical organizations), and uncertainties about reasonable risks and expectations all leave conservative organizational managers hesitant to make decisions. The design, implementation, and operation of effective, secure distributed systems are still not well understood by many users or designers, nor are methods for the detection and control of intrusions. Management ignorance and uncertainties translate into delays in defining requirements for, procuring, and deploying modern health care information systems. Distributed system technologies, including security, need to be demystified, and managers must be educated about realistic goals, alternative solutions, and operational practices to take advantage of these tools. Only in this way can the health care industry improve its practices for protecting electronic health information.

5

Organizational Approaches to Protecting Electronic Health Information

Organizational policies and practices are at least as important as technical mechanisms in protecting electronic health information and patient privacy.[1] Organizational policies establish the goals that technical mechanisms serve, outline appropriate uses and releases of information, create mechanisms for preventing and detecting violations, and set rules for disciplining offenders. Though generally most effective in protecting against abuses by legitimate system users—insiders or trusted others— organizational policies and practices can also provide guidance for establishing mechanisms to protect against outside attackers.[2] In the health care industry, organizational policies and practices must properly balance patients' rights to privacy against the need for care providers to access relevant health information for providing care. Failure to do so can make patients unwilling to reveal sensitive health information to their providers or make such information too difficult to access when needed for care.

---

[1]Policies discussed in this chapter focus on maintaining the privacy of patient information. Health care organizations may have additional policies in place to protect the privacy of health care providers and of other information that the organizations consider confidential.

[2]Throughout this chapter, the term "user" is meant to include all employees with access to computing systems (whether full-time, part-time, temporary, or transferring), medical staff (including both admitting and referring physicians), contractors, vendors, students, and volunteers.

Creating a health care organization that is fully committed to safe-guarding personal health information is difficult. It requires managers and employees, both individually and collectively, to engage in an ongoing process of learning, evaluation, and improvement to create an environment—and an organizational culture[3]—that values and respects patients' rights to privacy. Managers must provide leadership by heightening awareness of privacy and security issues and by determining how the organization can achieve the most appropriate balance between access to electronic health information and patient concerns over privacy.[4] As front line caregivers, employees are responsible for the actual implementation of policies and procedures, and they may also participate in their development. Individual employees are the most likely sources of minor and accidental breaches of patient privacy, whereas inadequate policies or a lack of technical mechanisms are probably responsible for larger breaches.

As the committee's site visits attest, health care organizations have developed a number of policies and practices for protecting electronic health information. These include formal policies regarding information system security and patient privacy, formalized structures for developing and implementing policies and procedures, employee training practices, and procedures for monitoring and penalizing breaches of privacy and security policies. Nevertheless, additional progress needs to be made to improve organizational protections for electronic health information. Few, if any, health care organizations have developed an integrated approach to organizational managment that addresses all aspects of information security and patient privacy. Numerous obstacles must be overcome in order to provide organizations with the incentives and motivation to adopt stronger practices.

FORMAL POLICIES

Health care organizations have adopted a range of formal policies to outline their goals with regard to patient privacy and security. These include policies related to authorized uses and exchanges of health information and patient-centered policies that are intended to promote a stron-

---

[3] "Organizational culture" is a term inclusive of the values, norms, understandings, and experiences of organizational employees, as well as patients, payers, and purchasers.

[4] Valuing patient privacy does not follow from a proclamation by an organization's managers; values can be effective only when they are individually held. Some organizational researchers suggest that management should communicate facts about policies and then demonstrate a strong commitment to that policy through their own behavior. See Larkin, T.J., and Sandar Larkin. 1996. "Reaching and Changing Frontline Employees," *Harvard Business Review*, May-June, pp. 95-104.

ger relationship between patients and providers with regard to maintaining patient privacy. Both the content of policies and the approach used to develop them play a large role in ensuring that employees abide by them. Policy documents are most effective when designed as easily accessible, ongoing reference materials and when introduced at the start of employment and referred to regularly in training and other internal communications.

Policies Regarding Information Uses and Flows

Policy statements regarding information uses and flows attempt to balance the need for providers, payers, researchers, and others to access health information against patients' desires for privacy. Overly restrictive policies, by making information inaccessible and leaving providers vulnerable to malpractice litigation, may interfere with providers' abilities to care for patients properly. Overly permissive policies may cause patients to lose confidence in the ability of the organization to protect sensitive data, making them reluctant to impart vital information. Notwithstanding common principles for balancing access and privacy, specific decisions may vary across organizations according to the size, structure, and types of care provided. Organizational culture also plays a strong role.

Policies regarding information use and flows tend to be formalized in specific policy documents on security, confidentiality, protection of sensitive health information, research uses of health information, and release of health information. They address both paper and electronic health records to avoid possible inconsistencies in the procedures employees follow for handling them.[5] Formally developed policies vary among organizations according to their internally developed risk assessments (Box 5.1).

Security Policies

Security policies describe an organization's philosophy and goals for user authentication and access control, as well as data reliability, availability, and integrity. Effective policies generally include a description of the organization's risk assessment and assign responsibility to individu-

---

[5]At present, the electronic medical record is an attempt to transfer paper records into electronic form. Over time, the electronic medical record will incorporate content such as images and sound that cannot be stored in paper form. Modern telecommunications may also provide the opportunity to capture content not previously considered part of the patient record, such as teleconferences and on-line consultations.

BOX 5.1
Risk Assessment

In conducting a risk assessment, organizations consider the following:

- The value of the assets being protected.
- The vulnerabilities of the system: possible types of compromise, including the vulnerability of users as well as systems. What damage can the person in front of the machine do? What about the person behind it?
- Threats: do adversaries exist to exploit these vulnerabilities? Do they have a motive, that is, something to gain? How likely is attack in each case?
- Risks: the costs of failure and recovery. What is the worst credible kind of failure? Possibilities are death, injury, loss of privacy, fraud.
- The organization's degree of risk aversion.

These considerations must be balanced against:

- Available countermeasures (both technical and nontechnical); and
- Their direct costs and (indirect costs of implementation).

SOURCE: Computer Science and Telecommunications Board, National Research Council. 1991. *Computers at Risk: Safe Computing in the Information Age.* National Academy Press, Washington, D.C., adapted from pp. 59-60.

als, committees, or departments for developing specific procedures and mechanisms by which the policy is to be implemented (see Chapter 4).

Confidentiality Policies

Confidentiality policies describe the overall approach to be taken in balancing access to information against protection of information. They may also provide details about the organization's risk assessment so that readers can understand why certain behaviors and procedures are important.

Organizations often have a number of datasets that management considers confidential: individual health information, financial data, business plans, employee files, outcomes research, and so on. Each of these datasets may be considered corporate assets and their disclosure may result in a financial disadvantage or loss to the organization. Although this perspective can provide strong incentives for protecting health information, health data are qualitatively different from proprietary corporate information and entail unique risks and liabilities. Confidentiality policies are most effective if they recognize the unique concerns associated with health information and provide adequate protection.

As a matter of policy, most provider organizations allow physicians to access the records of all patients within the institution; this approach ensures that information will be available when needed for care, and it is technically simpler than more restrictive approaches. Committee members also observed alternative approaches that, although perhaps not widely applicable or scalable, more narrowly restrict access to health information. For example, some organizations allow all staff and admitting physicians unrestricted access to all patient files, but limit the access privileges of referring physicians to their patients of record. This approach enables an organization to restrict the access of physicians with only occasional need to access the system, but still leaves unrestricted the large number of physicians who regularly have patients admitted or seen at the organization.

Other organizations allow physicians unrestricted access to information about their current patients, but allow access to other records only if a specific and documented need arises. In such cases, the information system can prompt the caregiver to type in the reason for access or to select the reason from a list. Common reasons such as "consult requested by primary care provider" or "emergency care" are supplied on the screen, as well as a fill-in-the-blank option. An e-mail notification of the access can be sent automatically to the primary care physician for review.[6] Inappropriate access is deterred when system users understand that their actions will be recorded and reviewed and that sanctions can be applied for violating patient privacy. This system balances the need for restricted privileges against emergency or unexpected needs for access without requiring burdensome or time-consuming behavior.

Policies to Protect Sensitive Information

Most health care organizations have policies that establish special protections for sensitive information such as mental health records, HIV status, drug and alcohol treatment, as well as the health records of celebrities and other widely recognized persons. Protection of some information is guided by state or federal legislation (see Chapter 2); other protection is provided voluntarily by individual organizations. Some sites visited by committee members either kept sensitive information apart

---

[6]"E-mail notification of access" is but one feature of an audit trail system that records details about information access. See the Chapter 4 section "Audit Trails" for further discussion of the topic.

from the rest of the health record or provided greater security for the entire health record if it contained sensitive information.

Paper-based health records are often accorded special protection by simply locking them up (in the office of the director of medical records, for example) when not in active use. None of the sites the committee visited had tried to mimic this system with their electronic records (by removing records from the system entirely or by limiting access to a few, select providers); but in some sites, the information system generated additional prompts or warning screens, informing users of the sensitive content of the records and reminding them that audit logs maintained a record of all accesses to patient records. Users were required to type in their log-on ID or password again as acknowledgment that they had read and understood the warning. Users reported that the warning screen causes them to pause and think again about their reasons for accessing the record and that this approach successfully deters unnecessary attempts to access records of celebrities (which are often motivated as much by curiousity as by medical need).

Other organizations have chosen not to include sensitive information in the electronic medical record; rather, the medical record contains a note stating that additional information is available from another physician or department. While effective in removing sensitive information from the record, this approach does not fully protect privacy. If a note in the record states that additional information is available from the psychiatric department, for example, any user accessing the primary record can infer that the patient is being treated for psychiatric problems. Furthermore, some sensitive information must be kept in the main record to ensure adequate care. Medication lists are typically included in electronic medical records because of the need to avoid prescribing drugs that interact with one another to cause an untoward effect. For this reason it is impractical to withhold certain drugs from the electronic record even though they may be a nearly unambiguous indication of a sensitive condition (e.g., a positive HIV diagnosis).

Alternatively, some sites indicated that the contents of the electronic medical record are a matter of ongoing negotiation between patient and provider. In some cases, the most sensitive (and sometimes most critical) information is left out of the formal record when patients expressed concerns over privacy. In these instances, providers often maintained handwritten notes kept in a separate file, raising issues (and concerns) about what constitutes the real record.[7]   Withholding information from the

---

[7]Separate, handwritten records are not always a guarantee that they will remain confidential between a patient and his or her physician. See *Consumer Reports.* 1994. "Who's Reading Your Medical Records?," October, pp. 628-632.

health record has implications for care: it is often difficult to determine a priori what information will be important to later delivery of care. Separate, or secret, records can hinder care in emergency situations and may have legal implications if a record is subpoenaed. But physicians may choose to negotiate with patients over the content of the record if it means the patient will continue to seek care.

A small number of health care organizations allow patients considerable control over access to their health information. One particular organization that works with people with AIDS allows patients to determine which providers are allowed to access their records and which portions of the record they are authorized to see. Another organization that manages a state health program (but does not provide care) lets patients (or clients as they are referred to by the site) allow only their case worker to access patient records. As these examples demonstrate, technology is available for creating fine-grained access controls by the patient, but these controls appear to be applicable only in a limited set of circumstances with a narrow patient base. It does not appear that these practices could be applied easily to health care organizations with more diverse, transient patients who receive episodic care.

An alternative approach that is used successfully by some health care organizations is to avoid segregating sensitive information from the rest of the medical record and to instead improve the security of the entire, integrated medical record through the use of well-designed authentication procedures, access controls, audit procedures, and other mechanisms. The goal of this approach is raise the level of protection for *all* health information, not just sensitive information. The advantage of this approach is that it ensures the medical record contains all available information that a care provider may need to make sound decisions about a patient's condition or treatment plan. The disadvantage is that it might require overly burdensome security practices for some applications or make organizations reluctant to offer some types of information services. For example, organizations may not want to allow Internet access to its clinical information systems if such access will be provided to the full medical record. In such cases, however, it may be possible to relax the security on some limited subsets of data. For example, one organization allows physicians to access information on patients in the intensive care unit from home or during travel. Screens show current laboratory results and vital signs for patients in the intensive care unit, but refer to them only as, for example, the "37-year-old, white male in bed 4." This information is insufficient to identify the patient to a casual intruder but is enough for a physician familiar with his or her patient profiles. Such a process works well in a controlled setting such as the intensive care unit, where a limited number of patients are under close and frequent supervision. The committee believes that this approach serves to protect patient privacy well in similarly controlled settings while allowing care providers easy and immediate access to vital information, but it probably would not scale well to larger units.

Policies on Research Uses of Health Information

Organizations (especially those linked to either a medical school or a medical research program) must also develop policies to guide researchers in procedures for maintaining patient privacy while using health information. These policies should contain a clearly formulated statement that defines "intended use" and defines identifiable versus aggregate data access. Procedures for removing identifying factors need to be clearly specified for both the paper and the electronic medical record and for record abstracts or audit material. The standard (and generally acceptable) pathway for review of requests for research access to medical record information is through an organization's institutional review board (IRB), whose members evaluate the potential for patient risk as a result of granting access (Box 5.2). Sites visited by committee members had experienced no instances of researcher abuse of confidentiality policies, and their IRB mechanisms seemed to function well to reduce such risk.[8]

Policies with regard to institutional review boards also may include procedures on how to obtain IRB approval, a clearly specified statement of IRB function and protocols, and lists of its regularly scheduled meetings and reviews. One site visited by committee members had a particularly well-developed process that required researchers from outside the organization to seek collaborative relationships with staff physicians and obtain approval for an appointment as a visiting scientist before applying for access to the organization's patient health information. This site would not allow external researchers to copy records in any form for their own use; paper records needed to be audited or read on-site. Visiting scientists were allowed only copies of aggregate datasets with all identifiers removed, and then only with the approval and knowledge of their collaborating on-site researchers. The information system was defined formally as an organizational resource to be carefully guarded and preserved; outsiders were allowed access only if they agreed to apply for, and could achieve, internal legitimization.[9] Staff from this site routinely

---

[8]Of note is the fact that a great deal of internal research activity is not reviewed by an IRB or any other oversight committee. Such studies include reviews of quality of care, surgical outcomes, and resource utilization. It is not clear the extent to which identified patient information is necessary for this research, but because the studies do not relate directly to patient care, there arise issues of confidentiality in the use of patient information.

[9]Establishing a formal affiliation between a researcher and the organizational owner of patient information better enables an IRB or other specified group to monitor compliance with the originally approved research protocol.

BOX 5.2
Institutional Review Boards

The Institutional Review Board (IRB) system and process rests on two sets of federal regulation. The first requires that any conduct of research on human subjects by agencies of the U.S. government or supported by the U.S. government must receive IRB approval before proceeding; the underlying model is that of government-supported biomedical subjects. Second, the Food and Drug Administration requires research involving human subjects and new drugs or devices to be approved by an IRB. Regulations require IRBs to have at least five members, one of whom is from outside the institution. IRBs review the benefits and risks to subjects of proposed research and the importance of knowledge that may be reasonably expected to follow, and examine the process by which investigators explain relevant issues in order to obtain informed consent from the subjects.

SOURCES: Rosnow, Ralph L., Mary Jane Rotheram-Borus, Stephen J. Ceci, Peter D. Blanck, and Gerald P. Koocher. 1993. "The Institutional Review Board as a Mirror of Scientific and Ethical Standards," *American Psychologist* 48(7):821-826. See also Edgar, Harold, and David J. Rothman. 1995. "The Institutional Review Board and Beyond: Future Challenges to the Ethics of Human Experimentation," *Milbank Quarterly* 73:489-506.

---

reviewed published research articles to detect possible violations of the organization's policy.

Policies Guiding Release of Information

Defining the circumstances under which health information may be released and to whom is a first step in ensuring that patient privacy is not violated by inappropriate disclosure. Common elements of policies on release of health information include defining (1) who is authorized to release information, (2) who is authorized to receive information and under what conditions, (3) the form and scope of information that may be released, and (4) the circumstances under which additional patient consent is required.

Organizations may track releases of patient information by retaining in the permanent health record the signed authorization form (when one is required), records of what information was released, the date of release, to whom it was released, and the signature of the employee who released the information. This record keeping creates an audit trail if unauthorized disclosure is suspected.

Patient-centered Policies

A number of practices have been developed to help improve communications between patients and providers regarding the collection, use, and dissemination of health information. These practices make individuals more aware of their rights regarding their health records, the consent they give for using and disseminating health information, and the existence of electronic medical records. In the short term, greater patient awareness of data issues and their rights may create liabilities for the organization: better-informed patients are more likely to hold organizations responsible for protection of their health information. In the long term, however, organizations using these practices are more likely to evolve cultures that value the protection of health information and avoid potential liabilities, fostering more open and candid interactions between patients and providers and increasing the likelihood that relevant data will be available for patient care.

Patient Bill of Rights

Some organizations have developed or adopted a patient bill of rights that outlines clearly the relationship between patient and provider; states the patient's rights to privacy and confidentiality; and outlines state and federal laws, regulations, and standards guaranteeing those rights. For example, it may describe a patient's right to view the audit trail related to a hospital stay or the procedures by which a patient may review the contents of his or her health record and correct information he or she believes is inaccurate.[10] The name and telephone number of a contact person within the organization who is responsible for patient complaints with regard to privacy and security (e.g., an information security officer) is included for patients who believe that their rights have been violated. The patient bill of rights is coordinated with forms authorizing disclosure of individually identifiable health information to ensure compatibility between the two documents.

Authorization Forms

Disclosure authorization forms inform patients of the existence of the electronic health record and describes the policies and procedures in place

---

[10]In most cases, a patient statement correcting information contained in the health record is submitted as an amendment to the record rather than a substitution. This method resolves concerns that a patient's view may differ from that of a care provider.

to protect patient privacy. They provide patients with information on what parts of the record are usually shared with other providers or insurance companies or are used for internal management purposes (over which the patient has no control) and request authorization from patients for any other intended uses. They may also provide patients with a statement of their rights to access their health record.[11] At least one of the sites visited by committee members had recently completed an extensive review of its forms during which legal terminology had been removed, making the language clearer and more understandable, and the forms had been translated into the languages common to the organi-zation's patient population. This site had worked with patient representatives to test their ability to understand the forms.[12] Coordinating a patient bill of rights with a disclosure authorization form can further enhance the relationship between provider and patient by helping to establish mutual understanding and trust.

Access to Records and Audit Logs

Many health care organizations allow patients to review their own health records and to correct or amend records, as necessary, through a formal process. Some states require provider organizations to allow such access; other states make no such provision and individual institutions are free to set their own policy. Organizations that allow patients to access their own health records find that it can not only help ensure the integrity of the information contained in the record, but can help patients better understand its content and sensitivities. Most have developed formal policies for access; some allow patients to review records only in the presence of one of their employees who can both explain the content of the record and ensure that it is not altered. Other health care organiza-

---

[11] The legal right for a patient to review or copy his or her own medical record is explictly granted only in about half of the states (see Jeffrey, Nancy Ann. 1996. "Getting Access to Your Medical Records May Be Limited, Costly—or Impossible," *Wall Street Journal*, July 31, pp. C1 and C21).

[12] The term "informed consent" is commonly used in the health care community to refer to authorizations that patients give for health care and related activities. Privacy advocates have expressed concern, however, that authorizations often are not "informed"; nor do they represent "consent." They claim that, at the very least, the person signing the form should understand its contents. The patient should understand also what information will be shared, with whom it will be shared, and how it will be used. Representatives of the health care organization should take steps to test whether or not the patient understands: for example, has the patient said no to any part of the form? Has the patient requested more information? Informed consent is both difficult to measure and difficult to test.

tions will, upon request, analyze the audit logs of accesses to a particular patient's record. This practice is useful in detecting alleged violations of confidentiality. Though exposing health care organizations to possible legal action, such reviews can, in the long run, help reduce patients' suspicions and provide the motivation for organizations to develop strong measures for protecting patient information.

ORGANIZATIONAL STRUCTURES

Formal organizational structures are needed to develop, implement, and enforce policies regarding privacy and security. These structures take on a variety of forms, depending largely upon the nature and culture of the institution in which they will operate, and serve as a focal point for both management and technical issues related to the safeguarding of privacy and security in paper and electronic medical records. Institutions with strong organizational policy tend to have well-defined structures with clear lines of responsibility. They typically include groups charged with developing policy; offices or departments for implementing policy, and structures for granting access privileges to users of the institution's information systems. A fourth structure—the institutional review board—is discussed above in the section titled "Policies on Research Uses of Health Information."

Policy Development Process

Health care organizations develop privacy and security policies in many different ways: by a small cadre of senior executives, by a committee process that solicits input from across the organization, or by some combination of the two. Committee members saw a range of approaches during their site visits. One site developed policy primarily within senior management, with limited input from department heads, users, and patients. Another organization used committee structures for all policy development activities. Policy developed by a small group of high-level executives has the advantage of being less time-consuming than a committee process and inherently carries with it the authoritative power of management. At the same time, it is becoming increasingly understood that employee input into policy decisions increases the likelihood of acceptance and effective implementation.[13]

Most sites visited for this study developed policy by committee. These

---

[13]Kanter, Rosabeth Moss, David V. Summers, and Barry A. Stein. 1986. "The Future of Workplace Alternatives," *Management Review* 75(7):30-33.

committees went by different names (for example, health records, confidentiality, security, and information systems management) in different
institutions and had different reporting structures. Some reported directly to upper management; others were part of a larger medical records
committee. Regardless, committee composition is generally broad and
may include members with knowledge of user needs and behavior (e.g.,
health information managers, nurses, physicians, admitting managers,
human resources managers, and patient relations representatives), technical experts on the organization's information systems, lawyers, and patient representatives.[14] Upper management often assists committee members by helping them to define a scope of work that complements rather
than duplicates other organizational efforts and by requesting clear mile-
stones for committee accomplishments. Using a committee structure to
develop policy can be time-consuming and subject to delay; one site that
had adopted a consensus decision-making style to ensure buy-in found
the advantage offset by its time-consuming nature. Employees at this site
commented also that committee memberships were often large (with
members from each interested department) and subject to turnover, which
further contributed to delay. Nevertheless, ensuring appropriate representation of interests is key to developing sound policy.

Structures for Implementing Policy

Once policies have been developed and approved, procedures are
needed to translate their intent and goals into everyday practices, which
may vary somewhat across departments. Whether or not the same individuals or committees that developed the overarching policy take on or
delegate the task of developing procedures is not as important as ensuring that authority and responsibility for implementation are clearly assigned. Responsibility derives from accountability: unless management
makes it clear that responsibility has been delegated, no one may assume
responsibility, and employees may not know where to go with questions
or problems. Accountability is particularly problematic in organizations
in which committees formulate policies but individuals or departments
are charged with policy implementation.

Several of the sites visited by committee members had designated an

---

[14]Another goal of broad committee membership is to include both system users and
system designers. Input may be sought from the broader population as well by means of
"comment boxes" into which users can drop suggestions for policy changes or system
redesign. Also important is ensuring that the concerns of patients are met. In the sites
visited by the committee, organizations often charged legal counsel with representing patient concerns. Other options include community representatives on key committees or
active solicitation from the community via open meetings or annual surveys.

information security officer to handle the design, implemention, and evaluation of confidentiality and security policies; this person also was the single point of contact for patients or employees to report incidents or concerns related to inappropriate disclosure of health information. In these organizations, the information security officer was a technically knowledgeable manager who reported directly to the chief information officer and served on relevant policy-making committees. For example, one information systems committee developed policy that said protecting patient privacy required the use of audit trails. That organization's information security officer then developed procedures that included a description of how often an audit trail should run, what information should be recorded, and what actions a patient should take in order to review audit trail data. Some organizations may add the duties of an information security officer to those of an existing employee; larger organizations may establish a new position or even a department.

Another role for which an information security officer may be held responsible—and one that requires a strong technical background—is risk assessment. Of the sites visited by committee members, few had formal programs for evaluating the presence and magnitude of various threats to the organization's health information. This is an ongoing activity that, at a strategic level, informs the policy development process, as well as the allocation of financial resources.

An information security officer needs a clear charter of authority from management to avoid conflicts with other departments. For example, an investigation into a breach of policy committed by an employee may become derailed if personnel from human resources believe employee discipline falls solely under their aegis. Although authority should clearly fall in one place or another, cooperation among departments with similar charters supports the overall goal.

Structures for Granting Access Privileges

The process by which users are granted or denied access privileges to an information system is key to maintaining the security of that system. Procedures are necessary for granting access to new users, changing access privileges for users who take on new responsibilities or transfer to different departments, and terminating access privileges for users who resign or whose employment is terminated. New users need privileges granted quickly in order to perform their jobs; transferring or temporary employees need access privileges updated to reflect their changing responsibilities; users who lose or forget their log-on IDs or passwords need a rapid response from the granter of privileges; employees who are terminated should have access privileges revoked promptly. Typically, responsibility for granting or denying access privileges is assigned to information systems personnel, human resources personnel, supervisors, others appointed by management, or some combination of the above.

The structure for granting access privileges may be centralized or distributed. In a centralized model, information systems personnel usually grant the privileges approved by others. The advantage of this approach is that workers in the information systems department understand system requirements and the levels of access defined for various user roles; they are centrally located and easily contacted. The disadvantage is that they may not understand requests that stray from standard guidelines. Similarly, human resources personnel are responsible for administering new hires, transfers, and terminations and need to be closely involved in granting access privileges, but they are not close enough to the practical needs of health care providers to appraise unusual, but legitimate, requests for access.

Several sites used a more distributed model. In one instance, corporate vice presidents assigned authority to supervisors or department heads in various areas to grant access to particular databases or applications. Employees requested access privileges from the relevant authority and demonstrated their need to know. Supervisors understood job responsibilities (and, in fact, assigned them) that crossed standard role-based access privileges and, thus, were able to evaluate the request. In emergency situations, workers could be granted access to clinical systems from a head nurse. This model has the advantage of assigning responsibility for certain sets of data to the employees most likely to understand legitimate requests for access. Having a variety of access granters helps ensure that someone will be readily available in all but the most unusual circumstances. A disadvantage that may be demonstrated is a lack of coordination among access granters that can lead to the system being vulnerable to nontechnical activities undertaken by individuals with an intent to deceive. For example, unless the access granter is scrupulous about checking the legitimacy of requests, someone may pretend to need access when, in fact, no real need exists.

Another site used a decentralized system of data stewards and custodians. Data stewards are responsible for particular data sets. They are typically department heads, division chairs, or principal investigators on research projects who are knowledgeable about the content of the data sets and can make appropriate decisions about its protection. Data stewards are formally charged to (1) recommend mechanisms and practices for protecting the data; (2) communicate control and protection requirements to data custodians (see description below) and system users; (3) coordinate with the information systems department to authorize access to particular sets of data (e.g., laboratory results or surgical notes);

(4) monitor compliance and periodically review control decisions;[15] and (5) review security violations and report them to the appropriate manager.

Data custodians are information systems personnel responsible for implementing security procedures established by the data steward, including audit trail, system backup, and disaster recovery tasks, as well as granting access privileges to system users (e.g., a data steward authorizes a request for access and passes the operational task on to a data custodian). Custodians supply the stewards with audit trail data or other system warnings about unusual or inappropriate activity. Finally, data custodians generally detect and respond to violations of policy and procedure and weaknesses in security measures. They coordinate with data stewards to propose changes to policies and technical mechanisms to enhance security.

A system of data stewards and custodians divides the management of information into pieces that can be handled easily and assigns responsibility for its security to the managers and technical personnel most likely to recognize unusual or inappropriate activity. It distributes decision-making authority to those who best understand the confidentiality concerns associated with the data and can best identify those with a need to access the data. Decentralization also encourages a greater number of system users to value the security of electronic health information by holding them responsible for it. On the other hand decentralization requires an effective coordination strategy to avoid inconsistent implementation of policy. A clear process must be in place to ensure that data stewards are identified, notified of their responsibilities, and given proper training. In one site that used this approach, many people were unaware that they were data stewards, and other employees did not know to whom to go with questions about particular datasets. Mechanisms are also needed to allow data stewards to share information on good practices.

EDUCATION AND TRAINING

Education and training programs are critical to an organization's attempt to protect patient privacy and information security. Formal training programs seek to educate system users about existing policies and

---

[15]For example, a data steward may periodically review user accesses that have been granted over a predefined period (e.g., 30 days) and follow up with information systems personnel or even users whose access privileges appear inappropriate. A data steward may also review portions of audit trail data that track users accessing their datasets and investigate patterns of unusual usage.

proper procedures so that they can incorporate them into everyday behaviors. They can also help employees internalize the value of patient privacy. Training users before allowing them access to health information reinforces management's commitment to protecting patient privacy. Both formal and nonformal training programs can help workers understand their responsibilities for protecting information and learn the procedures they must follow to do so. A variety of education tools and policy instruments, such as confidentiality agreements, can serve this role.

Training Programs

Most health care organizations have formal classes or programs to educate employees about patient privacy and system security. Many provide such training in an orientation session before they are given access to patient information. Similarly, refresher courses serve to remind long-time users about existing policies, update them on changes, and discuss strategies for real-life situations that they may encounter on the job. Transferring employees also need training to help them understand how their new position changes their responsibilities with regard to privacy and security.

Several of the sites visited by committee members provided training on a regular basis at both the organizational and the departmental levels in order to convey general policies as well as the particular requirements of a user's department.[16] To make the abstract message more concrete, a special effort was made to discuss specific circumstances encountered in particular departments that might involve or threaten patient privacy. Some sites also held interdepartmental workshops or in-service sessions to discuss practical applications of confidentiality policy. Because some participants may have scheduling limitations, training options often include flexible delivery formats, widely varying schedule choices, and contingency plans that may include one-on-one sessions for extreme cases.

Training medical staff to use the information system and to safeguard data privacy or security poses special challenges for a number of reasons. In addition to their busy schedules, physicians often have a variety of relationships with health care organizations: they may be employees,

---

[16]An alternative approach offers training based on job role to recognize that various user groups access electronic medical records in different ways (e.g., look at different information) or to varying degrees (e.g., 1 to 2 times a day versus 80 to 100 times a day). For example, a class for nurses may cover privacy and security issues more comprehensively than a class introducing volunteers to the admitting department (who probably will not have access to clinical information).

they may be under contract, or they may simply admit or refer patients to a health care facility. Several of the sites visited by the committee noted that the historical role of physicians made it difficult to require them to attend training; at least one site proposed requiring even nonemployee physicians to participate in training activities in exchange for access to the facility's computer system. Physicians often view training as a disruptive and unnecessary intrusion into an already busy schedule with competing demands, but organizations that tie training tightly to policy on privacy and security can both emphasize its value and accommodate cultural and scheduling conflicts (Box 5.3).

Most sites using a standard training module for new employees (lecture, handouts, film) reported that such modules are not at all effective in either capturing physician interest or imparting lasting information. To help spark physician interest in the importance of data security, a different form of system training is needed. Innovative training methods have been evaluated in studies on changing clinical practice behaviors and may be of use for training in confidentiality and security as well.[17] Among the types of techniques that might be incorporated in confidentiality and security training is the use of grand rounds in health provider organizations in which cases or vignettes involving inappropriate disclosure of health information are examined in detail and adjudicated by medical staff. Physicians could also be encouraged to enroll in continuing medical education courses focused on confidentiality and security issues. Another possible technique used effectively by drug companies—detailing— might be customized to present one-on-one training to individual physicians or small groups of physicians. No matter which training techniques are developed for physicians, it is imperative that the leadership of the medical staff, both chairs of clinical departments and the chief of staff, be involved in their development and act as champions of and models for patient privacy.

Nonformal Training

Often, the most effective training occurs in spontaneous or unintended ways. One of the sites visited by committee members relied more on socializing new employees into an organizational culture that stressed the "highest moral, ethical, and legal standards" than it did on orientation and training programs. Nevertheless, this practice can backfire unless the

---

[17]Soumerai, S., and J. Avorn. 1990. "Principles of Educational Outreach to Improve Clinical Decision Making," *Journal of the American Medical Association* 262:549-556.

organization has taken care to develop a culture that values privacy and security as much in practice as on paper. New employees seeking to fit in emulate their coworkers, but senior employees who have fallen into bad habits may pass their habits along to others. Similarly, if physicians routinely discuss patients over lunch in the cafeteria, ward clerks may soon come to understand that privacy is just another word in the policy manual.

In addition to the training and education employees receive about their day-to-day responsibilities, they need to participate in activities that support and encourage organizational learning. Organizational learning refers to the willingness of employees both individually and collectively to examine policies, procedures, and resulting behaviors and their effect on patient privacy. This happens only in organizations where the dominant culture stresses the importance of employee involvement in policy development and procedural evaluation. Similar to efforts toward total quality management, organizational learning involves a constant process of questioning the underlying goals of a policy, the effectiveness of procedures in appropriately guiding policy into practice, and the degree to which actual behavior reflects procedures. Managers and employees individually and collectively take responsibility for asking whether patient needs (both in terms of health care delivery and in terms of privacy) are being met and what changes would more effectively support that goal.

The cultural environment supports organizational learning by either valuing questions or discouraging them. One site visited by committee members denied the probability of breaches of patient privacy on the grounds that "nobody here would do that." By failing to acknowledge that individuals can (either through accident or malice) fail to protect patient privacy, the organizational culture ensured that changes in policy and practice were unlikely to occur. These "organizational defensive routines"[18] are patterns of behavior that prevent employees from having to experience embarrassment or threat (e.g., confrontation over behavior that led to breaches of patient privacy) and, at the same time, prevent them from examining the nature and causes of that embarrassment or threat. In the absence of mechanisms to the contrary, new employees are likely to emulate the conduct of experienced personnel—whether or not that conduct is in compliance with established organizational policy.

Educational Tools

A variety of tools may be developed to support or enhance formal

---

[19]Argyris, Chris. 1994. "Good Communication That Blocks Learning," *Harvard Business Review*, July-August, pp. 77-85.

BOX 5.3
Training Physicians in Privacy and Security

The difficulty of involving physicians in effective information system training is symptomatic of the changing basic professional norms and values in the practice of medicine. Most models of the medical profession are careful to distinguish between the content of medical work (the actual practice of medicine) and the terms and conditions of medical work—the organizational, employment, and contractual arrangements defining the relationship between the physician and the clinic, group, hospital, health maintenance organization, preferred provider organization, or health system where medical care is delivered.[1] Although physicians continue to exert considerable control over the content of their work, there has been a marked erosion of physician control over the terms and conditions of that work. Most physicians who work within managed care settings are familiar with this development; however, they are still somewhat uncomfortable with the reality of modern medical work defined as both the process of delivering care and the process of creating, maintaining, and transmitting information about that care. Medical notes and patient charts traditionally have been someone else's responsibility; now, physicians must encounter the information system directly, and must then be responsible for how information is created, used, and safeguarded. Physician resistance to accepting this responsibility may be owing to the fact that responsibility for such charting tasks historically has been associated with clerical staff. Physicians are likely to define information processing tasks as part of the terms and conditions of medical work, rather than as part of the core of medical work. Once that historical association is weakened and the core of medical work is redefined as both care process and information process, resistance may also weaken.

The first and most obvious way to help overcome such resistance is to work toward revision of the medical school curriculum so that training in information systems and the importance of data security is more than cursory. Medical school curriculum changes are slow to develop and spread; thus, this type of solution can be expected only in the long term. Currently, many managed care organizations complain that primary care physicians hired at the postresidency level often lack experience with information systems and must be given extensive in-house retraining.[2]

Within managed care organizations and health maintenance organizations it is possible to directly impose information system training and responsibility for data

---

training programs. These include attractive pamphlets, enhancements to computer systems, self-study modules available for use in the computer training center or to take home, and posted reminders in elevators and cafeterias.

An organization's information system may be designed to educate users as to possible breaches of confidentiality. Described earlier was a screen used at one site that appeared whenever users accessed sensitive information. The screen contained text reminding users that they were accessing sensitive information and asked the user if the action was justified. Another common option is to display an abbreviated version of the

security as part of a physician's performance review. Management within such settings usually has more direct control (either employment or financial) over physician practice behavior. It has also become more common in these settings for physician performance reviews to include statistical profile information on practice behavior,[3] thus more closely aligning the observable outcomes of health information systems with the practice of medicine.

A somewhat less coercive strategy that could be used in any medical care organization—whether managed care or traditional, freestanding or system affiliated—has to do with linking the credentialed status of physicians to the need for an internal role model on information system security. Of the hundreds or thousands of employees in modern health care organizations, only physicians still possess the status associated with the medical credential and the Hippocratic oath, especially its entreaty "to do no harm." Physicians could use their status within health care settings to set an example regarding the importance of health information privacy and security that should be mirrored by all other employees with access to the information system. Physician training that taps into this role may be found more acceptable and more meaningful, both to physician members and to the organization as a whole.

---

[1]Hafferty, Frederic, and Donald Light. 1995. "Professional Dynamics and the Changing Nature of Medical Work," *Journal of Health and Social Behavior,* extra issue, pp. 132-153.

[2]Vanselow, Neal. 1996. "New Health Workforce Responsibilities and Dilemmas," pp. 231-242 in M. Osterweis et al. (eds.), *The U.S. Health Workforce: Power, Politics and Policy.* Association of Academic Health Centers, Washington D.C. See also Fulginiti, Vincent. 1996. "The Challenge of Primary Care for Academic Health Centers," pp. 247-252 in *The U.S. Health Workforce: Power, Politics and Policy,* M. Osterweis et al. (eds.). Association of Academic Health Centers, Washington D.C.

[3]U.S. Department of Health and Human Services, Agency for Health Care Policy and Research. 1995. *Using Clinical Practice Guidelines to Evaluate Quality of Care,* Volume 1. U.S. Government Printing Office, Washington, D.C., March. Also, Murrey, Katherine, Lawrence Gottlieb, and Stephen Schoenbaum. 1992. "Implementing Clinical Guidelines: A Quality Management Approach to Reminder Systems," *Quality Review Bulletin,* December, pp. 423-433.

confidentiality policy every time a user signs onto the information system. Unless organizations change the appearance of these screens on a regular basis, however, they are unlikely to be effective. For example, changing the presentation or the content will catch a user's eye.

Self-study computerized modules may offer additional opportunities for nonformal training. These could be offered across departmental desktop machines or at a central location such as the human resources department.

At least one of the sites visited by committee members developed a special pamphlet to present the organization's confidentiality and security policies. Because it was short and visually attractive, this pamphlet captured users' attention in a way that a chapter in a larger policy manual could not. With the word "confidentiality" prominently displayed on the cover, it included the following information:

- *A summary of the organization's confidentiality philosophy and reference to the policy.* Users were referred to specific sections of the main policy manual for further information related to what information was to be considered confidential, procedures to follow for ensuring confidentiality, and disciplinary actions that would follow breaches of policy.
- *References to relevant statutory and regulatory requirements.* A synopsis of relevant law reinforced the organization's policy and emphasized that confidentiality was not simply an organizational requirement.
- *References to specific functions of the information system designed to reinforce policy.* The pamphlet described how (in that state) users' ID and password combinations constituted their legal signature, informed users of the existence of audit records, reminded them they would be held accountable for the files they accessed, and described a function that allowed users to look up accesses to their own record compiled when they themselves were patients of the organization.
- *A reminder to users about patients' rights and users' responsibilities.*

The pamphlet was distributed to new users during orientation and was readily visible in work areas. The organization stressed that a "person's medical record exists in several formats, including the electronic one."

Additional measures can be implemented to reinforce policy manuals. Of the sites visited by the committee, at least one had developed a video to reinforce key concepts of the organization's policies on patient privacy and security and help make them stand out from information on benefits, recycling, and cafeteria hours. New employees watched the video during orientation before a system ID and password were issued. Unlike a commercial product with anonymous actors, senior executives in the organization introduced policy concepts, demonstrating management's commitment to maintaining the confidentiality of health information. The video included examples that helped personalize violations to employees. Actor-employees in the video re-created instances where patient privacy had been breached; many of them seemed initially innocent, reinforcing the message that even good intentions can lead to unintended consequences. In one example, an employee was disciplined for accessing another employee's electronic health record to obtain a mailing address for a get-well card. The organization was successful in delivering the message because it presented examples to which employees could relate.

A key factor in reinforcing organization policy is the practice of re-training every year. Annual installments remind employees that policy is in place to guide their behavior; they also allow an organization to educate employees about changes that have resulted from statutory or regulatory changes, procedural changes, and changes in the threat environment. At least one site visited by committee members had sections to be marked off on the employee performance review form that verified the employee's attendance at training and his or her viewing of the confidentiality video.

In addition to a formal policy guide, periodic memos and newsletters were circulated to employees by some sites in order to provide regular reinforcement and to make a tangible addition to the employees' knowledge base. Information on changes in the data system were distributed routinely, and the ongoing policies were regularly reinforced.

User Confidentiality Agreements

In addition to informing employees of the organization's expectations with regard to keeping health information confidential, organizations need to hold them responsible for their behavior. Of the sites visited by committee members, several required any individual accessing the information system to sign a form verifying that he or she had read, had understood, and was committed to the organization's confidentiality policies.[19] In keeping with other ongoing efforts, employees were required to sign this agreement during the initial orientation session and annually thereafter at the time of their performance review. Confidentiality agreements may also be used for nonemployees who have access to health information; these can include contract workers, vendors, physician's office staff, students, temporary workers, and volunteers. See Box 5.4 for a sample confidentiality agreement developed by the Computer-based Patient Record Institute (CPRI).

SANCTIONS FOR BREACHES OF CONFIDENTIALITY

The most effective response to either internal or external violations of confidentiality policies follows from disciplinary sanctions described in

---

[19]The Computer-based Patient Record Institute advises that all health provider organizations will benefit from developing confidentiality agreements. These include hospitals, physician offices, home health agencies, pharmacies, nursing homes, and others. See Computer-based Patient Record Institute (CPRI). 1996. *Sample Confidentiality Statements and Agreements for Organizations Using Computer-based Patient Record Systems,* Work Group on Confidentiality, Privacy, and Security. CPRI, Schaumburg, Ill., May.

BOX 5.4
A Sample Access and Confidentiality Agreement (Physician)

As a physician with privileges at (HEALTHCARE ENTITY) (hereinafter referred to as "Physician"), you may have access to what this agreement refers to as "confidential information." The purpose of this agreement is to help you understand your duty regarding confidential information.

Confidential information includes patient/member information, employee information, financial information, other information relating to (HEALTHCARE ENTITY) and information proprietary to other companies or persons. You may learn of or have access to some or all of this confidential information through a computer system or through your professional care to patient/members.

Confidential information is valuable and sensitive and is protected by law and by strict (HEALTHCARE ENTITY) policies. The intent of these laws and policies is to assure that confidential information will remain confidential—that is, that it will be used only as necessary to accomplish the organization's mission.

As a physician with access to confidential information, you are required to conduct yourself in strict conformance to applicable laws and (HEALTHCARE ENTITY) policies governing confidential information. Your principal obligations in this area are explained below. You are required to read and to abide by these duties. The violation of any of these duties will subject you to discipline, which might include, but is not limited to loss of privileges to access confidential information, loss of privileges at (HEALTHCARE ENTITY), and to legal liability.

As a physician, you must understand that you will have access to confidential information which may include, but is not limited to, information relating to:

• Patient/members (such as records, conversations, admittance information, patient/member financial information, etc.),
• Employees (such as salaries, employment records, disciplinary actions, etc.),
• (HEALTHCARE ENTITY) information (such as financial and statistical records, strategic plans, internal reports, memos, contracts, peer review information, communications, proprietary computer programs, source code, proprietary technology, etc.), and
• Third party information (such as computer programs, client and vendor proprietary information, source code, proprietary technology, etc.).

Accordingly, as a condition of and in consideration of your access to confidential information, you promise that:

1. You will use confidential information only as needed to perform your legitimate duties as a physician of patient/members affiliated with (HEALTHCARE ENTITY). This means, among other things, that:

• You will only access confidential information for which you have a need to know;
• You will not in any way divulge, copy, release, sell, loan, review, alter or destroy any confidential information except as properly authorized within the scope of your professional activities as a physician of patient/members affiliated with (HEALTHCARE ENTITY); and
• You will not misuse confidential information or carelessly care for confidential information.

2. You will safeguard and will not disclose your access code or any other authorization you have that allows you to access confidential information. You accept responsibility for all activities undertaken using your access code and other authorization.

3. You will report activities by any individual or entity that you suspect may compromise the confidentiality of confidential information. Reports made in good faith about suspect activities will be held in confidence to the extent permitted by law, including the name of the individual reporting the activities.

4. You understand that your obligations under this agreement will continue after termination of your privileges as a physician, as defined in this agreement. You understand that your privileges hereunder are subject to periodic review, revision, and if appropriate, renewal.

5. You understand that you have no right or ownership interest in any confidential information referred to in this agreement. (HEALTHCARE ENTITY) may at any time revoke your access code, other authorization, or access to confidential information. At all times during your privileges as a physician, you will safeguard and retain the confidentiality of all confidential information.

6. You will be responsible for your misuse or wrongful disclosure of confidential information and for your failure to safeguard your access code or other authorization access to confidential information. You understand that your failure to comply with this agreement may also result in loss of privileges to access confidential information, loss of privileges, and to legal liability.

[space for signature follows]

_____

NOTE: CPRI points out that any organization initiating the use of a similar agreement should seek the advice of legal counsel.
SOURCE: Computer-based Patient Record Institute (CPRI). 1996. *Sample Confidentiality Statements and Agreements for Organizations Using Computer-based Patient Record Systems,* CPRI Work Group on Confidentiality, Privacy, and Security. CPRI, Schaumburg, Ill., May.

formal policy statements. Sanctions complement confidentiality and security policies by establishing penalties for violating them. If a policy is violated and no response follows, the validity of the structure to protect patient privacy is nullified. If appropriate sanctions are applied, but only irregularly, after a long delay, or with little impact on perpetrators, the structure is severely undermined, and its legitimacy is suspect.

Breaches of confidentiality and security policies originating from external sources may require assistance from local or federal law enforcement personnel, and organizations may seek redress through the courts. Breaches originating from internal sources may be dealt with in a variety of ways.

Although both types of breaches are potentially disastrous, internal breaches are more amenable to organizational sanctions. In fact, many industry leaders believe that the internal threat is far more dangerous and prevalent than the external threat. The chief executive officer of the firm that markets one of the leading Internet firewalls was quoted recently as saying: "It's ironic, because 80 percent of security breaches are internal—internal security is more important than perimeter defense. The outside world seems scarier, but the inside world is more dangerous."[20] The existence of clearly specified sanctions and well-understood procedures for their implementation are important signals to employees. Several practices appear to preserve the effectiveness of the structure as it relates to internal breaches of confidentiality.

Clear policies are needed for disciplining employees who violate confidentiality and security policies. Many organizations distinguish between intentional and unintentional violations by defining a policy of incremental discipline. Such a policy acknowledges the difference between intentional or malicious behavior and violations that result from carelessness or unintentional actions (e.g., leaving a computer terminal logged on). Organizations might provide an oral or written warning to an employee for a first or minor offense, suspend an employee for a second or greater offense, and terminate employment for major or repeated violations. A policy of "zero tolerance" that is used by some organizations states that all breaches will have swift and appropriate consequences, no matter by whom or for what reason the breach occurred. If evidence shows that a breach has occurred and a guilty party can be identified, disciplinary action follows quickly and in accordance with the signed confidentiality agreement.

The committee observed a range of established sanctions and disciplinary actions at the sites it visited. At least one site had no written sanctions and dealt with violations on a case-by-case basis. Other sites described sanctions in policy documents but were uneven in applying them; for example, clerical employees may have been fired, but physicians were "cautioned" behind closed doors. Another site had a clearly stated and observed zero-tolerance policy; employees were treated similarly throughout the hierarchy, and the organization publicly announced the results of its investigations and disciplinary actions.

Effective policies depend on consistent and evenhanded implementation. Inconsistently applied penalties encourage employees to believe that they can avoid them. Unevenly applied penalties can cause friction among staff and undermine confidentiality and security policies.

For sanctions to act as an effective deterrent, employees must know

---

[20]*Information Week*, Vol. 3 (June 1996), p. 12.

that they exist and will be implemented. Descriptions of sanctions should be included in confidentiality and security policies. Organizations that make disciplinary actions public can find that this serves as a strong example of management's willingness to enforce policy; one site visited by committee members, however, cautioned that such an approach can create an atmosphere of mutual suspicion and violate employees' own rights to privacy.

Organizational culture is an important source of the norms regarding appropriate information access and use, and is one source of guidance for the definition of appropriate sanctions for violations of accepted norms in these local situations. Most of the organizations visited by committee members had spent little time on the delineation of appropriate sanctions for the abuse or inappropriate use of health care information; it appears that industry standards in this area have yet to be developed. Given the high level of mutual suspicion among health care providers, their employing organizations, and associated financial organizations, it is not yet clear how useful it would be to publicize widely the ways infractions of information rules and policies are handled.

IMPROVING ORGANIZATIONAL MANAGEMENT: CLOSING THE GAP BETWEEN THEORY AND PRACTICE

Each of the sites visited by committee members indicated a strong interest in and concern for patient privacy but often failed to have adequate written policies or to demonstrate behavioral compliance with existing policies. Typical of inadequate or incomplete policies was the lack of clear definition of what was meant by a lapse in security or a breach of patient privacy—or of what these meant in the context of the health information systems maintained by the organization. Employees disagreed over whether problems referred to mere episodic technological breakdowns or to truly malicious incidents. Moreover, there was a lack of specificity as to who was responsible for these events when they did occur and what constituted an appropriate disciplinary response.

Further, few organizations had formal mechanisms for modifying confidentiality and security policies. Committee members observed several well-documented policy statements and some excellent protocols for the training of organizational employees. Not only do these concrete and clearly specified policies make it easier to interpret and enforce confidentiality and security rules and procedures, but they also serve as reinforcements to existing cultural values and perceptions. The organizations that appear to have moved toward stronger cultural supports for confidentiality and security controls are those in which the values, policies, and procedures have come from the very top of the organization. Yet, without scheduled, annual reviews of these policies and procedures and their continued reinforcement by management, there is risk that these policies will no longer have relevance or impact within the organization.

Implementing an Integrated Security and Confidentiality Management Model

Although each of the organizational strategies described in this chapter was observed in at least one site visited by committee members, no site had implemented all and some had implemented very few. Sites often demonstrated a lack of clear leadership on the part of management; thus, employees were uncertain of what to do or where responsibility lay. The committee observed instances in which employees had made isolated efforts to improve practice within their departments, but without sufficient authority and management support, these efforts remained limited in scope and had little impact on the overall organization.

As organizations expand their boundaries they need to develop a comprehensive program to ensure that the message of commitment to patient privacy is pervasive and implemented in policies, procedures, and everyday behavior. Such a model includes an overall vision and goal statement, specific policy development, training, and provisions for disciplinary action.[21] It enables employees involved in developing policies and procedures to understand the ultimate goal of their efforts, as well as how those efforts complement parallel efforts elsewhere within the organization. Through early, careful, and explicit planning, management serves as a coordinator and helps ensure that policies are not in conflict, lines of authority are clear, and gaps in security are avoided.

A model system would operate both top-down, with management outlining broad policy goals, and bottom-up, with employees developing local solutions, to form a matrix of communication, participation, and cooperation. The committee believes that the practices described in this chapter represent mechanisms by which patient privacy can be better protected; implemented together they may be described as an integrated management model for protecting patient privacy.

---

[21]A comprehensive program includes written policies, standards, training, technical and procedural controls, risk assessment, auditing and monitoring, and assigned responsibility for management of the program. See Computer-based Patient Record Institute (CPRI). 1996. *Guidelines for Managing Information Security Programs,* Work Group on Confidentiality, Privacy, and Security. CPRI, Schaumburg, Ill., January.

Overcoming Obstacles to Effective Organizational Practices

Organizations face a number of obstacles in developing an integrated approach to confidentiality and security. These obstacles derive from a lack of internal and external incentives that can motivate an organization to dedicate the resources necessary to establish the full range of policies, practices, and structures necessary to ensure stronger protection of electronic health information. These obstacles include resource constraints, competing demands, a lack of focus on information technology, and cultural constraints.

Lack of Public or External Incentives

As discussed in Chapter 2, there are few legislative or regulatory requirements that address patient privacy directly. Few existing controls provide adequate recourse for patients whose privacy has been breached. In addition, there have been relatively few broadly publicized events that have rallied public interest in privacy issues. In many cases, events have focused on a celebrity or public official, reinforcing the belief that the broad population of patients is unlikely to be harmed. At least one of the sites visited by committee members believed little would happen if its entire database of patient information were made public.[22]

As the committee conducted its study, it has become apparent that although most health care organizations express a commitment to patient privacy, their actual practice is somewhat different. This does not vary remarkably from other commercial and industrial organizations. Policy making in business organizations with regard to the confidentiality and security of information may generally be characterized as "drifting" on a path of incremental "policy by least steps" until these organizations experience a direct threat and an effort is made to respond to or repair the damage.[23] Although business organizations may have written policies on confidentiality and security, these policies may no longer be relevant to current business practices and activities.

At the same time, changes to policies made in reaction to events in the external environment can result in policies being too narrowly focused.

---

[22]Recent events, however, may have begun to change this perception. See Tippit, Sarah. 1996. "A New Danger in the Age of AIDS," *Washington Post*, October 14, p. A4. See also Brelis, Matthew. 1995. "Patients' Files Allegedly Used for Obscene Calls," *Boston Globe*, April 11, pp. 1 and 6.

[23]Smith, H. Jeff. 1993. "Privacy Policies and Practices: Inside the Organizational Maze," *Communications of the ACM* 36:105-122.

Examples of external catalysts include state and federal legislation but often are the result of business concerns, regulatory problems, lawsuits, or—most important—poor public relations. Business concerns grow out of heightened interest in keeping information from falling into the hands of competitors. They may also be the result of industry pressure to adopt a more stringent code of ethical conduct. Decisions to release or withhold information can leave organizations open to suits by disgruntled patients, employees, employers, and nonaffiliated health care providers. Several sites reported increased impetus in their policy-making process after a lawsuit had been filed or a breach reported in the media. Many sites also reported an increasing number of concerns expressed by individual patients that led to review (and sometimes revision) of existing policies.

Resource Constraints

Maintaining patient privacy is an important objective for health organizations, but it must compete with numerous other budgetary demands. As employees at sites visited by committee members indicated, health care organizations spend about 2 percent of their annual budget on information systems and about 2 percent of that on information security. Information security is often among the first items to be cut in the face of budgetary pressures. As in other industries, health care organizations do not act until a gross breach of patient privacy has occurred. According to one expert, sales of security products in the financial industry rise sharply after a breach is reported in the media, but drop off just as sharply after about 10 days. Several sites visited by committee members indicated that protection of health information does not serve as a market differentiator, and managers were therefore unwilling to allocate funds to support it.

Competing Demands

Many health care organizations are deep in the throes of developing integrated delivery systems (IDSs) by acquiring clinics, other hospital sites, and specialty practice groups, as well as retail pharmacy sites, long-term care facilities, and related organizations.[24] Merging multiple organizations is a highly complex and often confusing process that stretches the resources of organizational members.[25] As management focuses on high-

---

[24]According to Deloitte and Touche LLP (*U.S. Hospitals and the Future of Health Care,* Philadelphia, 1996), 71 percent of U.S. hospitals either belong to an IDS or are participating in the development of one. IDSs are emerging as the predominant organizational model in today's health care environment.

[25]Although much has been written in industry periodicals, the popular press, and aca-

level negotiations and financial agreements, it is often unable to focus also on the details of how the resulting organization will function. Establishing IDS management processes for confidentiality is secondary or tertiary to formalizing the merger or acquisition, negotiating the make-up of a management team, cutting redundancy and positioning for market share, and developing a single health information system. From observations made during the committee's site visits, it is clear that the integration of systems, policies, cultures, and procedures is usually left to be worked out after the merger discussions have been completed. Organizations often keep separate information systems functional until more comprehensive business integration takes place; issues concerning systemwide information security are considered later on a catch-up, patch-up basis.

As IDSs form, they begin to wrestle with the problem of redesigning their information systems around multiple system platforms, home-grown technologies or software, legacy systems, and multiple distributed systems across multiple sites. Managers of IDSs must define the boundaries and relationships of the new organization. Among the questions to be resolved are the following: Who should have access to which parts of the data system? What is the relationship between employee users and nonemployee users? What are the philosophy and goals with regard to confidentiality and security for the new organization? Who decides these? What is the architecture of the merged information system? Who controls it? This is a process rather than an event, and beginning to work on it during negotiation of the merger or affiliation will ease the transition to a new organization. Employees who are presented with a fait accompli often resist change, and the resulting clash of cultures can seriously jeopardize the future of an organization.

Lack of Focus on Information Technology

Information management has become an essential component of the financial and managerial aspects of health care organizations, as well as of the provision of clinical care. Health care organizations are no different

---

demic journals on health care system mergers and strategic alliances, it is clear that the development and the process of alliance or merger are still poorly understood. The best work in health care administration and health services research is still based primarily on case examples (see Kaluzny, Arnold D., Howard S. Zuckerman, and Thomas C. Ricketts III (eds.). 1995. *Partners for the Dance: Forming Strategic Alliances in Health Care.* Health Administration Press, Ann Arbor, Mich.); industry consultants still present models based on ideas of courtship and marriage (see Kanter, Rosabeth Moss. 1994. "Collaborative Advantage: The Art of Alliances," *Harvard Business Review,* July-August, pp. 96-108).

than any other business enterprise in this regard, except that many are pressed to catch up with the state of the art and science of computer-based information systems.

Providers of clinical medicine have had mixed reactions to the information revolution. On the one hand, some lament the passing of an era of personal ties between patient and physician—one usually carefully documented in the handwritten paper chart of the provider. On the other, many recognize the advantages of standardized health records as continuity of care becomes more difficult and physicians increasingly practice in groups and often substitute for one another in caring for patients enrolled in health care plans. Health information databases have become the professional memories through which the continuity and quality of patient care can be ensured for individual patients over time. As organizations become larger and more complex, electronic health information systems become more important as a means of monitoring and controlling both the quantity and the quality of care. The purposes for which health information is collected and the ways in which it is used have much to do with the way information systems are viewed by users.

Cultural Constraints

Organizational culture can either enhance or impede the intended effect of information confidentiality and security policies because it reflects the values, norms, understandings, and experiences of organizational participants. Some health care organizations have never really accepted the idea of patients as organizational participants; hence, when matters of privacy and security are raised, discussion centers on the proprietary value of such information, not on the threats to individual patient's rights to privacy. Health care organizations are focused on providing care, not on providing security.[26] Accordingly, technology is valued inasmuch as it supports that goal and does so in a way that is convenient to caregivers. To the extent that mechanisms to support privacy and security are introduced, they are tolerated only if they are relatively transparent to the main goal. Health care providers often believe that security

---

[26]A recent study survey of information systems trends conducted by *Modern Healthcare* and Coopers & Lybrand indicated that improving managed-care capabilities was the driving force behind priorities over the next 24 months. Maintaining or improving the security of patient information did not appear as a concern. See Morrissey, John. 1996. "A Broader Vision: CIOs Shift Strategy to Look Beyond the Hospital," *Modern Healthcare*, March 4, pp. 110-113.

mechanisms are redundant, that members of the profession are well intentioned, and that they would never violate a patient's privacy.

With the advent of modern telecommunications and computing technology, almost any business enterprise draws upon a vastly expanded, even global, spectrum of information and personal contacts, which help to shape the culture of the organization itself. Most health care organizations have increasingly permeable boundaries, and it cannot be assumed that once the culture of privacy and security is established within the organization's walls, there are no other risks. As health care organizations form alliances and other vertical or horizontal linkages and as communications by these component entities increasingly use modalities such as the Internet, not only are the proprietary interests of these organizations put at risk, but patient-specific data are also more widely exposed. The awareness and concern that health care organizations exhibit with regard to these matters are, to a large extent, products of the organizational culture within which these issues are addressed.

Individual organizations take on a distinctive pattern of dealing with issues such as privacy and security. To some extent, the way these issues are addressed can reflect an organization's response to issues involving all aspects of technology. For example, an organization whose leaders have thought of computers and information technology as beyond human capacity to control may accept on blind faith the claim that, once programmed and made operational, computer-based information systems require little human monitoring or oversight. The more that global cultural influences are felt in contemporary organizations of all types, the less likely is it that any individual organization will be dominated by the influence of one or a few leaders who exert their personal stamp on everyday business dealings.

Organizations whose leaders and participants generally deny the possibility of violations of patient privacy (e.g., "It can't happen here," or "We've never had a serious incident before") may engender a culture that essentially acts as a blinder to these issues. This represents one of the most important, and frequently observed, impediments to the adoption and effective implementation of risk reduction policies and structures. Yet, the cultural supports for an initiative involving privacy and security may constitute an essential ingredient for its success. Unless organizational leaders actively foster and nurture a security-enhancing culture, such policies and structures may be imposed but will have little influence on health care organizations.

6

Findings and Recommendations

Information technology offers many potential benefits to health care. Electronic medical records (EMRs) facilitate cost-effective access to more complete, accurate health data with which providers can make better decisions about patient care. Advanced communications networks can enable the sharing of data among distributed elements of integrated health care delivery systems and can enable telemedicine programs to overcome geographic boundaries between patients and providers. Electronic data processing techniques can enable managed care providers, health services researchers, and public and private oversight organizations to conduct more sophisticated analyses of health care utilization and outcomes. Electronic billing and administration systems may help reduce the administrative costs of health care. Computer-based decision support tools can help reduce variation in health care quality across providers, improve adherence to standards of care, and reduce costs by eliminating duplicative or nonefficacious tests and therapeutic procedures.

To obtain the benefits of electronic medical records, the nation must address and mitigate concerns regarding the privacy and security of electronic health care information. As the recommendations in this chapter describe, health care providers have to adopt a range of technical and organizational practices to protect health care information, and the health care industry will have to work with government to create a legal framework and proper set of incentives for heightening interest in privacy and security and for ensuring industry-wide protection of health information.

This chapter summarizes the committee's principal findings and presents recommendations for improving the privacy and security of health information. Although a number of the recommendations are directed specifically to electronic health information, many are equally applicable to the protection of paper records.

FINDINGS AND CONCLUSIONS

Finding 1: Information technology is becoming increasingly important in improving the quality and lowering the costs of health care; attempts to protect patient privacy must therefore center on finding ways to protect sensitive electronic health information in a computerized environment rather than on opposing the use of information technology in health care organizations. As the site visits conducted for this study attest, the shift to integrated health care delivery systems and managed care creates a growing demand for electronic health information and for data networks capable of transferring data within and across organizations. Electronic health information allows such organizations to better analyze data for such purposes as improving care, monitoring the quality of care, analyzing the utilization of health care resources, and managing health benefits. Care providers claim that the availability of health information on-line helps them enhance the quality of health care delivery, as well as its efficiency. Patients will see the advantages of integrating and sharing data across the institution as they begin to receive a greater proportion of their care within integrated delivery systems. The application of information technology to health care is expected to help reduce the cost of administering care.

Each of the organizations visited as part of this study has ongoing programs to expand the use of information technology for clinical care and administration; all reported positive benefits of such applications. As long as health care organizations continue to find value in these activities, whether by improving the quality or reducing the costs of care, strong incentives will exist to pursue them. Thus, although opposition to the use of electronic medical records may succeed in delaying their widespread adoption, in the long run expectations of enhanced quality and improved efficiency, combined with economic pressures, are likely to dominate. From a policy perspective, it therefore makes far more sense for the health care system to find ways to handle legitimate privacy and security concerns without foregoing the benefits of information technology.

Furthermore, properly implemented EMRs offer great potential for improving the security of health information and the privacy of patients. EMRs allow the use of technical mechanisms to either impede unauthorized access or deter potential abuses. For example, authentication and access control technologies can help ensure that access to health information is limited to people with a legitimate need to know. Audit logs can be used to keep a record of accesses to electronic records to detect abuse. Encryption can be used to keep health information secret as it is transmitted between users. Although none of these measures can guarantee absolute security, they provide a wide range of tools to ensure authorized access and use of health information. As a result, EMRs should not be viewed as a way of undermining patient privacy but as a means of enhancing patient privacy by improving the security of health information.

Finding 2: Health care organizations need to take a more aggressive approach to improving the security of health information systems in order to better protect electronic health information. Little is known about the extent of existing violations of privacy and security in the health care industry. Although some sites were aware of some cases in which authorized users had intentionally or unintentionally released health information inappropriately (from both electronic and paper record systems), the sites visited as part of this study reported no incidents in which outside attackers breached system security and produced large-scale violations of patient privacy. Most health care organizations therefore continue to perceive insider abuse as the primary problem to be solved; however, evidence from other industries indicates that organizations with Internet connections or other kinds of remote access (e.g., modem connections) are prone to outsider attacks.[1] As health care organizations put more information on-line and begin to transmit patient information electronically, they will have to ensure that adequate security protections have been developed to protect against new vulnerabilities.

Finding 3: Health care organizations have been slow to adopt strong security practices, due largely to a lack of strong management and organizational incentives; no major breach of security has occurred that has catalyzed such efforts. Thus, the information technology vendor community has not found a market for providing security features in health information systems. Although health care organizations are committed to ensuring privacy and security, the need to ensure access to information for the provision of care often works against having strong access controls and other security mechanisms. For example, hospitals often choose to allow physicians to access the health records of *all* patients, rather than

---

[1]According to one recent survey, nearly 25 percent of attacks against information systems that led to significant loss were due to outsiders. More than 50 percent of the survey's 1,320 respondents reported significant losses within the past two years. See Violino, Bob. 1996. "The Security Facade: Are Organizations Doing Enough to Protect Themselves? This Year's IW/Ernst & Young Survey Will Shock You," *Information Week,* October 21.

just their own, so that they can be certain to have access to needed information in an emergency. Concerns about the supposed inconvenience of using token-based authentication systems have led many health care organizations to rely on more convenient log-in IDs and passwords for authenticating users of health information systems. Even in cases in which security mechanisms would not necessarily impede provision of care, however, health care organizations have not always implemented strong security. Many organizations do not maintain audit logs of accesses to clinical information, nor have they developed tools or procedures for systematically reviewing the logs.

Lack of security results, in large part, from a lack of strong incentives to improve it. In the absence of a widespread, public catastrophe regarding information security, many health care organizations reported that they believe the risk of a major breach of security is low and that they could survive a major event without significant consequences. Without strong legislation or enforceable industry standards, few penalties will exist for lax security.[2] Although patients may sue organizations for damage resulting from alleged breaches of privacy, such suits appear to be infrequent and have not attracted much attention. Hence, most health care organizations have, to date, dedicated the vast majority of their information technology resources to expanding the functionality of health care information systems rather than to protecting the systems that are in place. System security does not improve the financial position of most health care organizations. In the more advanced organizations, security practices do not match those widely found in other industries, and in less advanced organizations, even elementary security practices have not been implemented. Several major vendors of health care information systems reported to the committee that lack of demand by health care organizations has stifled the supply of advanced security features in health care information systems. Since health care organizations do not reward them for including security features in their products, vendors have limited incentive to offer them.

Finding 4: Patients have important roles to play in addressing privacy and security concerns. Patient concerns and expectations often set the standard for health care organizations; health care organizations must anticipate and respond to such expectations in order to survive in an increasingly competitive environment. Thus, patients who are knowledgeable about (1) the consent they give providers to disseminate data,

---

[2]The Health Insurance Portability and Accountability Act of 1996 contains penalties for violation of privacy and security standards that have yet to be developed.

(2) overall flows of information within the industry, and (3) their legal and regulatory rights to privacy are in the long run an asset to an organization wishing to promote an internal culture that takes its privacy and security responsibilities seriously. Increasing the coupling between patients and provider organizations (e.g., through membership on key committees, messages sent to patients about privacy and security, and full disclosure of data flows) will ultimately benefit the organization.

Most patients and consumers are either unaware of or unconcerned about the uses to which their health records are put and the many organizations that possess their health information. Privacy and consumer advocacy groups that have a better understanding of data flows have yet to articulate a consistent position on privacy and security requirements and, until recently, have had limited influence on the legislative process. As a result, patients have little control over the ways in which information about their health is collected, used, or disseminated. For patients to feel comfortable providing personal health information to a care provider, they may need greater authority in helping to determine rules regarding the privacy of health information.

Finding 5: The greatest concerns regarding the privacy of health information derive from widespread sharing of patient information throughout the health care industry and the inadequate federal and state regulatory framework for systematic protection of health information. The current structure of the industry gives care providers, payers, pharmaceutical benefits managers, equipment suppliers, and oversight organizations a variety of incentives to collect large amounts of patient-identifiable health information (e.g., clinical data). The increasing emphasis on controlling costs and quality and on improving the marketing and sales of related products and services (e.g., medications) further boosts the economic value of such information. Although these data are collected for a variety of legitimate purposes, few controls exist to prevent such information from being used in ways that could harm patients or invade their privacy, and no national debate has occurred to determine what the appropriate uses of health information should be. The existing legal and regulatory framework for protecting patient-identifiable information forms a patchwork of protection that is insufficient in an age of increasing interstate data transfers and of health care delivery systems that span state boundaries.[3] Federal laws protect mostly data in the control of the federal government, while state laws provide inconsistent

---

[3]See Schwartz, Paul M. 1995. "The Protection of Privacy in Health Care Reform," *Vanderbilt Law Review* 48(2):310.

protection and often apply only to limited kinds of health information. In some instances, federal law facilitates the private-sector collection of patient-identifiable health information (e.g., the federal Employee Retirement and Income Security Act, or ERISA, allows self-insured employers to collect such information on their employees by preempting state laws). As a consequence, many organizations within the health care system are free to collect and use large amounts of patient-identifiable health information for purposes that suit their economic interests, and patients lack legal standing to bring suit against those they allege have breached their privacy. Data collected for one benign and stated purpose can be used for different, unstated purposes that may run contrary to the interests or understandings of the parties from which the data were collected. For example, self-insured companies that request patient data to monitor benefits programs have few legal constraints to prevent them from using such information in employment or promotion decisions.

In organizations that are subject to formal privacy protections, such as hospitals with mandatory institutional review boards that oversee research uses of health information (see Chapter 5) and government agencies subject to the Privacy Act of 1974 (see Chapter 2), privacy concerns seem greatly diminished. These types of structures appear to have been effective in ensuring uses of health information that are consistent with privacy concerns.

Finding 6: Within individual organizations, electronic health information is vulnerable to both authorized users who misuse their privileges and perform unauthorized actions (such as browsing through patient records) and outsiders who are not authorized to use the information systems, but break in with the intent of malicious and damaging action. Health care organizations have been working for many years to develop mechanisms for protecting health information (in both paper and electronic form) from abuse by authorized users, but they must continue to strengthen their protections by, for example, implementing auditing capabilities and strengthening disciplinary sanctions. As with other types of organizations, health care organizations will become more vulnerable to attacks by outsiders as they expand their networking activities. System vulnerabilities are not limited to breaches of privacy. If realized, the most serious vulnerability might well be a skilled individual with malicious intentions who can "crash" an important health information system and deny service to health care providers that rely on that system.[4]

---

[4]Of course, this is not unique to health information systems; the threat of outside attackers crashing a system is present in many other industries as well.

Finding 7: Adequate protection of health care information depends on both technical and organizational practices for privacy and security. Although no set of mechanisms can make organizations impervious to malicious attack or inadvertent breaches of security, a suitably crafted set of technical and organizational practices can be designed to protect health information effectively. Technologies such as tokens, log-in IDs, and passwords can be used to authenticate, or verify the identification of, users. Access control techniques can be used in combination with a well-managed information repository to limit the types of data that individual users can read, enter, or alter and the types of functions they can perform. Audit trails can record all transactions that access patient information. Encryption can be used to protect log-in IDs, passwords, databases, or information transmitted over open communications systems. Public-key cryptography tools can ensure information integrity, user authentication (for digital signatures and nonrepudiation), and audit trails. The use of these technical measures can provide reasonable security for most health care applications but does not guarantee invulnerability against all technical attacks.

Organizational policies and practices are at least as important an element of security. Organizations need explicit policies governing the privacy and security of health information. Practices and procedures flow from these policies. The health care industry employs millions of workers who routinely handle patient-identifiable information as part of their jobs. They have more opportunities to disclose information inappropriately than do outsiders, and their jobs are challenging and frequently changing. Organizational mechanisms are needed to ensure that employees, medical staff, contractors, and vendors properly protect health information. Policies are needed to specify the formal structures, ensure responsibility and accountability, establish procedures for releasing information and assigning access privileges, create sanctions for breaches of security at any level of the organization, and require training in the privacy and security practices of an organization. The culture of the organization—dependent on, but not necessarily determined by, its senior leadership—establishes the degree to which employees take their security and confidentiality responsibilities seriously. Commitment of organizational resources not only helps establish organizational culture but also ensures that funds are available for salaries of security officers and staff, for procurement of adequate technical security mechanisms (e.g., firewalls), and for studying vulnerabilities and required practices.

RECOMMENDATIONS

As the findings above indicate, attempts to improve the protection of health information need to address privacy and security concerns at both the organizational and the national or industry-wide levels. Organizations need to improve their internal mechanisms for handling health information, and the health care industry as a whole needs to improve its practices for controlling and enforcing systemic uses of health information. In the absence of strong business motivations and economic pressures to improve privacy and security, other forces may be necessary to promote change. These include industry-wide efforts to develop sound practices for protecting health information, initiatives to better educate patients about health data flows, or government regulation or legislation to provide patients with enforceable rights to privacy. Educating the public may also be an effective option for prodding organizational leaders to place a higher priority on privacy and security needs, though to date such efforts have not proved effective. Legislative initiatives have been stymied by an inability to achieve national consensus, and standards organizations are fragmented and lack sufficient authority to promulgate or enforce standards for privacy and security.

The recommendations below outline the roles of health care organizations, the health care industry, and government in improving privacy and security practices within individual health care organizations, creating the industry-wide infrastructure needed to develop and encourage adoption of stronger privacy and security practices, addressing systemic issues related to privacy and security, and ensuring research to meet future technical needs. To the extent possible, the committee has attempted to identify the organization or organizations best qualified to implement each recommendation. In some cases, private and public organizations will have to sort out their respective roles so as to make the best use of their strengths and resources.

Improving Privacy and Security Practices

As the site visits suggested, one of the obstacles to improving privacy and security in health care organizations is a lack of knowledge about the types of technical and organizational practices that are effective in protecting health information. No generally accepted set of practices exists against which organizations can compare their efforts, nor do specific standards exist. Guidelines such as these would help educate users about the types of practices that are available for protecting health information, would help ensure that health information is protected adequately within institutions, and would ensure some degree of uniformity across the health care system. Promulgation of a set of guidelines for standard practices might provide the incentive that organizations need to commit greater resources to the development of sound security strategies and would help vendors determine which types of mechanisms to build into their products.

Because health care organizations vary considerably in the types of information systems they deploy and the types of information they use in electronic form, as well as in the resources they can devote to system security, appropriate security practices are highly dependent on individual circumstances. It is therefore not possible to prescribe in detail specific practices for all organizations; rather, each organization must analyze its systems, vulnerabilities, risks, and resources to determine optimal security measures. Nevertheless, the committee believes that a set of practices can be articulated in a sufficiently general way that they can be adopted by all health care organizations in one form or another. Moreover, the committee believes that a general set of practices can be adopted at reasonable cost given the current state of technology.

Recommendation 1: All organizations that handle patient-identifiable health care information—regardless of size—should adopt the set of technical and organizational policies, practices, and procedures described below to protect such information. The set is not expected to serve as a benchmark for the industry but is envisioned as a framework for helping organizations determine how to improve privacy and security within their own institutions. These policies either could help health care organizations meet the standards promulgated by the Secretary of Health and Human Services as directed by the Health Insurance Portability and Accountability Act of 1996 or could inform the development of such standards. The penalties established by this act for violations of privacy or security standards may provide sufficient motivation for organizations to adopt these policies. External auditing firms could also play a role by evaluating privacy and security practices as part of their annual audits of health organizations. Although auditing firms are not empowered to enforce the use of these practices, auditors' assessments might provide insight into areas that need strengthening to avoid potential liabilities.

Specific implementation of these policies, practices, and procedures will vary from organization to organization, depending on individual circumstances, but each organization should adopt the full spectrum of recommendations to ensure that it addresses all aspects of security. The committee hopes that individual organizations will exceed as appropriate the requirements set out below in addressing privacy and security needs specific to their own sites. Although the committee did not calculate the cost of implementing the policies, procedures, and practices outlined below, each was observed in an operational setting and reportedly had been implemented at reasonable costs. These practices and procedures will not make health information systems invulnerable to all potential forms of misuse or abuse, nor can they guarantee that the privacy of health information will not be compromised. They would, however, go a long way toward minimizing potential abuse by authorized users (whether intentional or unintentional) and make outsider attacks more difficult.

Described below are technical and organizational practices and procedures that can be implemented immediately without too much difficulty or expense, as well as technical measures that could reasonably be taken in the future as the relevant technologies advance. In each case, the committee has attempted to identify approaches that take into account the specific requirements of health organizations (as opposed to organizations in other industries), balancing the need for privacy and security against the need for access in order to provide care. Each of the practices described for immediate implementation was observed to operate successfully in a health care setting. Of course, the implementation of these policies, practices, and procedures within individual health care organizations will have to be adjusted to accommodate the requirements specific to those institutions and to the various types of departments and settings within them. The demands of an AIDS clinic may be different from those of a large, urban hospital. The demands of a hospital's billing department may be different from those of an emergency room. Thus, although it may be appropriate to program a terminal in the billing department or on a physician's desk, for example, to log-off automatically after a specified period of time, it may not be appropriate for the terminal in an emergency room or an operating room to do so. Organizations will have to take these considerations into account as they develop plans for implementing the policies, practices, and procedures listed below to make sure that they adopt a strategy appropriate to their needs.

Technical Practices and Procedures for Immediate Implementation

Individual Authentication of Users. Every individual in an organization should have a *unique* identifier (or log-on ID) for use in logging onto the organization's information systems. This approach will make it possible to hold individual users accountable for their actions on-line and to implement access controls based on individual needs. Sanctions should be in place to discipline employees who share their identifiers or fail to log off their workstations. Where appropriate and not detrimental to the provision of care, computer workstations should be programmed to log off automatically if left idle for a specified period of time (though the period of time will have to be adjusted to accommodate local and departmental operations). Password discipline should be exercised, requiring users to change passwords on a regular basis and to select passwords that cannot be guessed easily. Procedures should be established to (1) revoke the identifiers of employees who leave the organization; (2) identify and revoke other unused identifiers as appropriate; (3) ensure that only legitimate users are granted access to the organization's information system; and (4) guarantee that authorized users can access needed information in emergency situations.

Access Controls. Procedures should be in place that restrict users' access to only that information for which they have a legitimate need. Ideally, such controls should be based on the needs of individual users, but in practice they may have to be based on job categories. Narrow job descriptions should be used, where possible, to allow more fine-grained control of access privileges. For example, job titles such as "doctor," "nurse," or "physician's assistant" provide less control than titles such as "cardiologist" or "emergency room nurse."[5] Any of the models discussed in Chapters 4 and 5 can be used for distributing access privileges. The committee recognizes that individual organizations will have to determine the appropriate job categories within their facilities and decide whether medical staff is allowed to access the records of all patients treated by the organization (which is often the case today) or only of patients under their direct care. Again, the proper balance between access and privacy will depend on the specific setting and on the need to ensure access to information in emergency situations.

Audit Trails. Organizations should maintain in retrievable and usable form audit trails that log all accesses to clinical information. The logs should include the date and time of the access, the information or record accessed, and the user ID under which access occurred. Organizations that provide health care services to their own employees should implement the capability for employees to conduct audits of accesses to their own health records. Although self-audits will not necessarily identify large numbers of inappropriate accesses to health records, they have proved to be a cost-effective way of raising employees' awareness and appreciation of privacy concerns in organizations that have deployed them. In addition, all organizations should implement procedures for

---

[5]It should be noted that the use of fine-grained access controls can exacerbate the difficulty of keeping the data in medical records organized so that they correspond with the access privileges of the users. A variety of software tools are under development to assist in managing this task (see Chapter 4).

reviewing audit logs both in response to requests from individual patients and through more formal means (e.g., random sampling). The goal of this practice should be to deter users from attempting to access information inappropriately rather than to detect a large percentage of actual breaches. All organizations (whether providers or others) should begin to plan for future implementation of more rigorous audit trails as described below in the section of practices for future implementation. One dimension of planning would be to demand that vendors provide information systems that support audit trails.

Physical Security and Disaster Recovery. Organizations should immediately take steps to limit unauthorized physical access to computer systems, displays, networks, and medical records. For example, computer terminals should be positioned and located so that they cannot be used or viewed by unauthorized users; unauthorized personnel should not have access to the locations in which records (paper or electronic) are stored. Procedures should be developed regarding paper printouts of electronic medical records and the destruction of printouts that will not be incorporated into the formal record. As part of their program for ensuring physical security, organizations should develop and implement plans for providing basic system functions and ensuring access to medical records in the event of an emergency (whether a natural disaster or a computer failure). These plans should be practiced not less than once a year to ensure that they provide rapid recovery and that staff are adequately trained. Disaster recovery plans should include regular backups of clinical information so that it can be restored if the primary data are destroyed or invalidated. Many organizations run daily, weekly, and monthly backups so that data can be recovered from both recent and archival files. Health care organizations should ensure that contractors used to transport and store backup tapes have adequate policies in place for safeguarding the information and protecting integrity. Backup tapes stored in off-site locations represent a significant vulnerability that is often overlooked. Backup tapes stored off-site should be subject to strong physical security to prevent unauthorized access or should be encrypted so that they cannot be read while they are being transported or stored.

Protection of Remote Access Points. Organizations must protect their information systems from attackers who try to gain entry through external communication points, such as the Internet or dial-in telephone lines. Organizations with centralized Internet connections should immediately install a firewall that provides strong, centralized security and allows outside access to only those systems critical to outsider users. Organizations with multiple access points should consider other forms of protection, such as TCP wrappers, to protect the host machines that allow external connections.[6]   Organizations should also require an additional, secure authentication process for users attempting to access the system from remote locations (e.g., those using home computers or portable computers). This should take the form of either encrypted or single-session passwords (see Chapter 4). Organizations that do not implement either of these approaches should allow remote access only over dedicated lines.

Many health care organizations currently protect their remote access points by using dial-back procedures[7] or by embedding the remote access telephone number in the software employed by remote users to establish a connection. The committee does not consider such approaches adequate for protecting remote access points and recommends against their use as substitutes for these other techniques. It recommends that information systems that are not protected by firewalls or by strong authentication mechanisms be disconnected from public networks and linked only to secure dedicated lines for remote access.

Protection of External Electronic Communications. Health care organizations need to protect sensitive information that is transmitted electronically over open networks so that it cannot be easily intercepted and interpreted by parties other than the intended recipient. To do so, organizations that transmit patient-identifiable data over public networks such as the Internet should encrypt *all* patient-identifiable information before transmitting it outside the organization's boundary. Any of several available encryption schemes will suffice. Organizations that cannot or do not meet this requirement either should refrain from transmitting informa-

---

[6]TCP wrappers protect individual server machines, whereas firewalls protect entire networks and groups of machines. Wrappers are programs that intercept communications from a client to a server and perform a function on the service request before passing it on to the service program. Such functions can include security checking. For example, an organization may install a wrapper around the patient record server physicians use to access patient information from home. The wrapper could be configured to check connecting Internet Protocol addresses against a predefined approved list and to record the date and time of the connection for later auditing. Use of wrapper programs in place of firewalls means that all accessible server machines must be configured with wrapper(s) in front of network services, and they must be properly maintained, monitored, and managed. See Venema, Wietse. 1992. "TCP WRAPPER: Network Monitoring, Access Control and Booby Traps," pp. 85-92 in *Proceedings of the Third Usenix UNIX Security Symposium*, Baltimore, Md., September.

[7]In a dial-back procedure, a remote user dials a specified telephone number to access the system. The system then hangs up and checks the caller's number against a directory of approved remote access telephone numbers. If the number matches an approved number, the system dials the user back and restores the connection.

tion electronically outside the organization or should do so only over secure dedicated lines.[8]   Policies should be in place to discourage the inclusion of patient identifiable information in unencrypted e-mail.

Software Discipline. Organizations should exercise and enforce discipline over user software. At a minimum, they should immediately install virus-checking programs on all servers and limit the ability of users to download or install their own software. Census software or regular audits can be used to ensure compliance with such policies. Current technological tools for checking software downloaded from the Internet are limited; hence, organizations will have to rely on organizational procedures and educational campaigns to protect against viruses, Trojan horses, and other forms of malicious software and to raise users' awareness of the problem.

System Assessment. Organizations should formally assess the security and vulnerabilities of their information systems on an ongoing basis. At a minimum, they should run existing "hacker scripts" and password "crackers" against their systems on a monthly basis. During their annual audits, external auditors should require each organization to demonstrate that it has procedures in place for detecting system vulnerabilities and that it conducts formal vulnerability assessments.

Organizational Practices for Immediate Implementation

Security and Confidentiality Policies. Organizations should develop explicit security and confidentiality policies that express their dedication to protecting health information. These policies should clearly state the types of information considered confidential, the people authorized to release the information, the procedures that must be followed in making a release, and the types of people who are authorized to receive information. They should clearly reference relevant state and federal legislation regarding the confidentiality of health care information.

---

[8]Organizations that prohibit the use of external communications systems to transfer patient-identifiable health information will have to recognize that users may attempt to find other ways to communicate information outside the institution, whether through floppy disks or printouts that can be scanned and entered into another information system. Other policies and practices (some of which are outlined below in this chapter) are needed to address such flows of information, although they will continue to be difficult to detect and prevent.

Security and Confidentiality Committees. Organizations should establish standing committees charged with developing and revising policies and procedures for protecting patient privacy and for ensuring the security of information systems. Small organizations that lack the resources or personnel for a formal committee should, at a minimum, designate a person or a small group of people to develop policy.

Information Security Officers. Organizations should identify a single employee to serve as a security officer who is authorized to implement and monitor compliance with security policies and practices and to maintain contact with national organizations that promulgate and enforce guidelines and standards regarding system security. The security officer should have tools available for implementing access and retrieval control mechanisms, as well as the firewall functions that control access and transmittal to remote locations. The information security officer need not be a full-time position in a small organization, but sufficient time should be invested to ensure adequate protection.

Education and Training Programs. Organizations should establish education and training programs to ensure that all users of information systems receive some minimum level of training in relevant security practices and knowledge regarding existing confidentiality policies. All computer users should complete such training *before* being granted access to any information systems.

Sanctions. Organizations should develop a clear set of sanctions for violations of confidentiality and security policies. Such sanctions should be applied uniformly and consistently to all violators, regardless of job title. Organizations should exercise zero tolerance in enforcing sanctions, ensuring that no violation goes unpunished. Sanctions should be established in relation to the seriousness of the violation. Organizations should terminate employees who willfully violate policy and should report such violations to appropriate licensing boards, where applicable. Negligent, rather than willful, violations of policy should be given lesser sanctions. Organizations should ensure that processes are in place for adjudicating all alleged violations of policy.

Improved Authorization Forms. Health care organizations should develop authorization forms designed to improve patients' understanding of health data flows and to limit the time period for which patients authorize the release of health information. These forms should be separate from other consent forms (e.g., those requesting consent to provide care), should inform patients of the existence of an electronic medical record, and should outline the policies and procedures in place to protect patient privacy. In addition, the forms should explicitly list the types of organizations to which identifiable or unidentifiable information is commonly released (e.g., insurers, researchers, and managed care companies). The forms should authorize the organization to release the specified information for a limited amount of time only, after which the organization must obtain new authorization from the patient. Attempts should be made to write the form in language that is accessible to the patient population.

Patient Access to Audit Logs. Health care providers should give patients the right to request audits of all accesses to their electronic medical records and to review such logs. As with access to patient records, providers may retain the right to share the audit log with patients in the presence of a provider employee who can explain the reasons for legitimate access. This practice not only will enable patients to ensure that their privacy has not been violated but will also help educate patients as to health data flows and perhaps create a more trusting relationship between patients and providers.

Security Practices for Future Implementation

The practices listed above are intended for immediate implementation in order to provide health care organizations with a minimally sufficient level of security in the current environment. Over the next several years, the security environment will change significantly as health care organizations move more health information on-line and begin to transfer more information electronically between users. In order to prepare for this new world and maintain adequate privacy and security, practices will have to evolve. Health care organizations will need to continue to invest in security technology.

The practices outlined below are intended to help the health care industry prepare for the future. In large part, the ability of health care organizations to implement the technical practices recommended below will depend on the general availability of the relevant technology. In some cases, availability will be a consequence of demands in markets including but not limited to health care (i.e., the general business market). In other cases, products will become available only if health care organizations demand them. In either event, health care organizations should start planning now to implement these practices in the future. They should begin to work with vendors to define the requirements of future health information systems so that the systems will be available when needed.

Strong Authentication. Health care organizations should move toward implementing strong authentication practices that provide greater security than individual log-on IDs and passwords. Authentication systems incorporating single-session or encrypted authentication protocols (similar to the Kerberos protocol described in Chapter 4) are expected to become available in some commercial products as early as 1997 and should be adopted shortly thereafter. Token-based authentication systems that require some sort of card, button, or badge in addition to a user password should also be adopted. Such systems are used widely in the banking industry today (automated teller machines are an example) and are being used experimentally in some health care organizations. Though more costly than a system using log-in IDs and passwords, the additional protection of token-based systems is likely to become necessary in health care organizations, and the price of tokens and readers is expected to drop over the next several years as their use expands in other industries.

Enterprise-wide Authentication. Organizations should move toward enterprise-wide authentication systems in which users need to log on only once during each session and can access any of the systems, functions, or databases to which they have access privileges. Such systems should be generally available in 2001. Because such a system concentrates security for many systems in a single authentication transaction, it must be used in conjunction with other technical and management practices that ensure good password protection.

Access Validation. Organizations that store, process, or collect health information should use software tools to help ensure that the information made available to users complies with their access privileges. It is often difficult to partition medical records in a way that closely matches the access privileges of different types of users. For example, doctors' notes can contain sensitive information that many users with access to clinical information have no need to know. Access controls themselves, whether based on job descriptions or sets of individual user privileges, provide no means of ensuring that the data retrieved by individual users contain no information that they are not privileged to see. Efforts are currently under way to develop tools that will check the information being transmitted to the user to detect and mask information that they have no need to know.

Expanded Audit Trails. Health care organizations should implement expanded audit trails. It is reasonable to expect that by 2001, all health care organizations should be able to maintain logs of all internal accesses to clinical information, especially if they begin to demand audit capabilities today.[9]   In the longer term, health care organizations should pursue the use of technologies and products that support interorganizational (i.e., global) audit trails that allow all patient-identifiable health information to be traced as it passes through the health care complex.   Examples of such technologies include the cryptographic envelopes and electronic watermarking technologies described in Chapter 4.   These technologies are still in their infancy and will require additional research and development to become commercially viable (see Recommendation 5).

Electronic Authentication of Records.   All health care organizations that use computerized electronic systems for order entry, discharge summaries, and other critical records should incorporate technologies for electronic signatures.   At a minimum, such systems should record the log-on identifier of the user that enters or modifies data in an electronic record. Such capabilities are possible today and should be incorporated into all new systems brought on-line after 1999.   Whether or not a cryptographic digital signature is used is not as important as the capability to identify the individual who enters or alters each element of information in the electronic record.   Organizations that wish to use such signatures to establish evidentiary trails admissible in a court of law must pay attention to the legal requirements of the states in which they operate.   This recommendation is not intended to support or undercut various existing or proposed digital signature laws at the state level, although the federal Health Insurance Portability and Accountability Act of 1996 mandates the development of standards for electronic signatures by February 1998.

Creating an Industry-wide Security Infrastructure

Although individual organizations can make considerable progress in improving patient privacy and the security of health information by implementing the policies, practices, and procedures outlined in Recommendation 1 above, additional efforts must be taken at the industry level to facilitate long-term advances in privacy and security.   To date, most health care organizations have attempted to assess the vulnerabilities of their electronic health information systems and to develop solutions in isolation, without benefiting from the experience of others.   Greater collaboration in both of these areas promises long-term improvements in privacy and security throughout the industry.

---

[9]A regulation to promote these audit trails could be structured to allow adequate time for the development of such systems and to avoid costly retrofitting by requiring only that information systems deployed by health care organizations after 1999 have the functionality necessary to support audit trails.

Recommendation 2: Government and the health care industry should take action to create the infrastructure necessary to support the privacy and security of electronic health information. The comprehensive protection of electronic health information would benefit from an industry-wide infrastructure that would develop and promote adoption of proven practices for protecting privacy and security and would facilitate greater sharing of security-related information among organizations that collect, process, and store health information. Many of these tasks are currently conducted in a fragmented manner, with little coordination between standards-development bodies and accrediting agencies or between organizations responsible for different sectors of the industry, such as hospitals, managed care organizations, and insurers. The committee believes that greater coordination of these disparate efforts would help address many of the systemic concerns about the privacy of health information and would provide clear leadership to individual health care organizations regarding the standards with which they should comply. While health care organizations have strong incentives to develop health care applications of national information infrastructure, they do not necessarily have strong incentives to improve privacy and security. The committee makes three subrecommendations described below to support this goal.

Recommendation 2.1: The Secretary of Health and Human Services should establish a standing health information security standards subcommittee within the National Committee on Vital and Health Statistics to develop and update privacy and security standards for all users of health information. Membership should be drawn from existing organizations that represent the broad spectrum of users and subjects of health information. The Secretary of Health and Human Services has already charged the National Committee on Vital and Health Statistics (NCVHS) with recommending standards for the security of electronic health information as called for in the Health Insurance Portability and Accountability Act of 1996. NCVHS should appoint a standing subcommittee that would monitor changing concerns regarding the privacy of health information and new approaches to protecting such information. Although a number of disparate organizations are currently attempting to develop standards for the security of health information systems and patient privacy (including the American National Standards Institute's Health Informatics Standards Board and its members, the Computer-based Patient Record Institute, and the American Health Information Management Association), none of these organizations represents the broad spectrum of users of health information as well as NCVHS does, and none has demonstrated clear leadership in setting and promulgating standards. The decentralization of standards-making activities has instead tended to impede the dissemination and application of standards in the health care industry.

The committee recommends that the health information security standards subcommittee be empowered to advise and offer recommendations to the Secretary of Health and Human Services regarding (1) uniform standards of privacy and security that would apply to all users of health information, whether providers, payers, benefits managers, or researchers; (2) exchanges of health information between and among health-related organizations; (3) limits on the types of health information that different types of organizations should be allowed to collect (e.g., determining how much information the insurance industry needs for fraud detection) and how long such information may be kept; and (4) acceptable and unacceptable uses of health information for different types of organizations. It should be formed as a standing committee that will develop revised standards as the uses of health care information change and new technologies become available.

Recommendation 2.2: Congress should provide initial funding for the establishment of an organization for the health care industry to promote greater sharing of information about security threats, incidents, and solutions throughout the industry. Little is known about the extent of violations of privacy and security in the health care industry, in part because the health care industry lacks a formal mechanism for sharing information about the types of attacks and breaches of privacy that organizations have experienced, and mechanisms for improving privacy and security. Establishment of an organization to facilitate information exchanges would provide a means for improving the security of health care organizations as they move into a more networked environment and would provide a sounder basis for making policy. As with the computer emergency response team (CERT Coordination Center) at Carnegie Mellon University, which facilitates information sharing among the Internet community, such an organization would allow sharing of effective technical practices for authentication, access control, encryption, and disaster recovery, as well as organizational practices such as consent statements, employee education, audit trail analysis, provision of access to referring physicians, definitions and enforcement of need-to-know scenarios, confidentiality committee structures, and policies and procedures for exchanging clinical data between disparate provider organizations. At a time when the industry is entering a period of rapid computerization and profound restructuring, and hence facing new problems, a forum for exchange of information has obvious benefits.

The organization, nominally called Med-CERT, would (1) acquire reports of security-related incidents at health care organizations; (2) define best practices for addressing common problems; (3) make recommendations to the health information security standards subcommittee regarding standards for securing health information systems; (4) define needed research; and (5) act as a liaison between the health care industry and the computer security community at large (including the CERT Coordination Center, the NASA Automated System Incident Response Corps, and international bodies). In order to facilitate the cooperation of health care organizations, the organization would have to take steps to ensure the confidentiality of incident information shared with it. To ensure a degree of visibility, Med-CERT should be established either within the federal government or as a private entity with strong links to a government agency such as the Department of Health and Human Services. Given the fiscal realities and existing priorities of the health care industry, Med-CERT will undoubtedly require funding from the federal government. Initial funding need not be large, perhaps just enough to support a dozen full-time employees.

Addressing Systemic Issues Related to Privacy and Security

Recommendations 1 and 2 (with 2.1 and 2.2) are geared toward promoting better policies, procedures, and practices within health care organizations for protecting patient health information. As noted in Chapter 3, the greatest concerns regarding patient privacy stem from the widespread dissemination of information throughout the health care industry and related industries, often without the knowledge or consent of patients. In many cases, this information can be used in ways that are perceived as detrimental to patient privacy and contrary to the interests of patients. The committee recognizes that privacy interests are only one consideration in the use of patient health information and acknowledges the existence of considerable controversy regarding the extent to which such practices should be allowed. Such controversy pits the economic interests of companies that use health information against those of patients. **Although the committee was not constituted with the range of expertise needed to render judgments and recommendations in this area, it calls attention to the existence of this conflict and emphasizes the need to determine how and to what extent greater control needs to be taken over these flows of information in order to protect patient privacy. Only when such questions are answered can policy be properly formulated.**

Recommendation 3: The federal government should work with industry to promote and encourage an informed public debate to deter-

mine an appropriate balance between the privacy concerns of patients and the information needs of various users of health information. The purpose of this debate should be to reach some general consensus about the balance that should be struck between privacy concerns and the demands of organizations for health information. Attempts will be needed to develop initial consensus about the central issues and the parameters of an acceptable resolution. To further this debate and provide opportunities for better informing the debate, the committee makes five subrecommendations.

Recommendation 3.1: Organizations that collect, analyze, or disseminate health information should adopt a set of fair information practices similar to those contained in the federal Privacy Act of 1974. These practices would define the obligations and responsibilities of organizations that collect, analyze, or store health information; establish enforcement rights for patients; and make the flows of health information more transparent to patients (Box 6.1).[10] It is expected that, at minimum, organizations that collect, process, or disseminate health information would disclose information describing the existence and nature of all individually identified health data they retain, the source from which the data are collected, and the types of organizations to which they regularly release the data. Such disclosure helps educate patients about the flows of health data and their rights in controlling those flows, thereby facilitating the discussion of privacy and security issues and the development of consensus. Personal awareness of privacy rights and potential abuses is one of the best countervailing pressures against the economic incentives that drive organizations to share information. Moreover, public awareness and concern may be an essential prerequisite to the passage of necessary legislation of any strength.

Recommendation 3.2: The Department of Health and Human Services should work with state and local governments, health care researchers, and the health care industry to establish a program to promote consumer awareness of health privacy issues and the value of health information for patient care, administration, and research. It should also conduct studies that will develop a series of recommendations for improving the level of consumer awareness of health data flows. Patients generally know less about the collection and uses of health information than do care providers, insurers, managed care organiza-

---

[10] See Schwartz, Paul M., and Joel R. Reidenberg. 1996. *Data Privacy Law: A Study of United States Data Protection.* Michie Law Publishers, Charlottesville, Va.

BOX 6.1
Major Provisions of the Federal Privacy Act of 1974

The Privacy Act of 1974 is designed to outline the responsibilities of federal agencies regarding the collection, use, and dissemination of personal information contained in their records systems. The act adopts the set of principles outlined by a committee of the Department of Health, Education, and Welfare in 1973 for protecting privacy:[1] (1) there must be no secret personal data record-keeping system; (2) there must be a way for individuals to discover what personal information is recorded and how it is used; (3) there must be a way for individuals to prevent information about them, obtained for one purpose, from being used or made available for other purposes without their consent; (4) there must be a way for individuals to amend a record about themselves; and (5) an organization creating, maintaining, using, or disseminating records of identifiable personal data must ensure the reliability of the data for their intended use and must take reasonable precautions to prevent misuse of the data. The Privacy Act specifically

• Gives individuals the right to access much of the personal information about them kept by federal agencies;
• Places limits on the disclosure of such information to third persons and other agencies;
• Requires federal agencies to keep logs of all disclosures, unless systems of records are exempt from the act;
• Gives individuals the right to request an amendment to most of the records pertaining to them if they believe the records to be inaccurate, irrelevant, untimely, or incomplete;
• Allows individuals to pursue disagreement and noncompliance with a civil suit in federal district court;
• Makes federal agencies responsible for collecting only relevant information about individuals, getting the information directly from the individual whenever possible, and notifying the individual at the time information is requested; and
• Requires federal agencies to publish reports in the *Federal Register* for each new or modified record system, outlining categories of records maintained, their routine use, policies on their storage and retrieval, and other agency procedures related to the use, disclosure, and amendment of records.

---

[1]U.S. Department of Health, Education, and Welfare. 1973. *Computers and the Rights of Citizens.* U.S. Government Printing Office, Washington, D.C.
SOURCE: Office of Technology Assessment. 1993. *Protecting Privacy in Computerized Medical Information*, OTA-TCT-576. U.S. Government Printing Office, Washington, D.C., pp. 77-78.

tions, researchers, and others who make use of the information. Having a neutral party like the Department of Health and Human Services, which is also involved in the development of standards for electronic data exchange, privacy, and security, take a more active role in educating patients may help improve patients' understanding of health data flows and generate a more informed public debate. Studies could examine the use of current public media such as magazines, community college-based seminars, and local news media as vehicles for informing the general public about these issues.

Recommendation 3.3: Professional societies and industry groups[11] should continue and expand their leadership roles in educating members about privacy and security issues in their conference discussions and publications. These are the primary organizations for reaching health care professionals who use health information. Although each already has some initiatives under way regarding privacy, such programs need to be given higher priority. These organizations, whose members have a strong interest in the use of patient information in a clinical setting, could work with privacy advocates and patient representatives to gain a deeper, more comprehensive view of patient concerns regarding privacy and would then be in a better position to develop sound recommendations in this area.

Recommendation 3.4: The Department of Health and Human Services should conduct studies to determine the extent to which—and the conditions under which—users of health information need data containing patient identities. Attempts to limit or control the flows of data to users not involved in the provision of care—whether through legislative or other means—will have to be based on a thorough analysis of the types of uses that different types of organizations have for health information. Secondary users make many claims that patient-identifiable data are necessary for legitimate uses such as fraud detection and benefits management. These claims originated at a time in which public concerns for privacy were far less intense than they are today and in which technologies to protect anonymity were far less developed. A fresh look to determine the minimum set of patient-identifiable data needed for these stated goals could result in a significant reduction of collected data that

---

[11]These include, but are not limited to, the American Hospital Association, American Medical Informatics Association, American Health Information Management Association, College of Health Information Management Executives, Healthcare Information and Management Systems Society, Computer-based Patient Record Institute, and American Medical Association.

are patient identified. It may be possible to use aggregated or anonymous data for certain applications. In other cases, such as some long-term medical research, identifiable data may be the only alternative. Understanding these different uses and the differing needs for patient-identifiable data will allow a more reasoned debate of patient privacy issues.

Recommendation 3.5: The Department of Health and Human Services should work with the U.S. Office of Consumer Affairs to determine appropriate ways to provide consumers with a visible, centralized point of contact regarding privacy issues (a privacy ombudsman). Consumers currently have limited avenues for seeking redress of alleged violations of privacy or for fully understanding their rights in this area. Although some hospitals employ advocates to act on the patient's behalf in addressing a variety of concerns, privacy is only one of a variety of problems that these patient advocates must address, and many other provider organizations have no one to counsel patients about their rights to privacy. Moreover, there is no obvious place for patients to lodge concerns regarding alleged breaches of privacy by organizations that are not care providers, such as insurers, benefits managers, and marketing firms. Consumers need a mechanism for learning about their rights and how they may seek recourse for violations of fair information practices, and they need to be protected from the possibility that their access to care may be jeopardized by exercising their established privacy rights. A privacy advocate appointed within the Department of Health and Human Services is ideally situated to work with the Office of Consumer Affairs to determine the type of ombudsman that would be appropriate for health privacy issues.

Several different models for a privacy ombudsman are possible, depending on the anticipated size of the need and the level of decentralization desired. For example, a national telephone hotline could be established to provide consumers a "one-stop shop" for guidance regarding means of seeking redress; state offices could be established to field complaints from patients and conduct investigations as necessary. Several state Attorney General's offices already have ombudsmen to address patient safety and rights in nursing homes and to accept complaints regarding insurance companies; their roles could expand to address issues related to patient privacy, by taking advantage of existing capabilities and infrastructure.[12]

---

[12]Institute of Medicine. 1995. *Real People, Real Problems: An Evaluation of the Long-term Care Ombudsman Programs of the Older Americans Act*, National Academy Press, Washington, D.C.

Together, the five subrecommendations in recommendation 3 are intended to promote a broad public debate over the ways in which—and the extent to which—privacy considerations should enter into the nation's attempt to determine ways of adjudicating the competing interests of consumers and various organizations in society (providers, employers, payers for health care). If the result of this debate is a decision that the privacy interests of consumers should weigh more heavily in this competition, several legislative options could strengthen the hands of consumers (Box 6.2).

Developing Patient Identifiers

The systemic issues relating to patient privacy are strongly related to the possible development and promulgation of a universal patient identifier. The Health Insurance Portability and Accountability Act of 1996 directs the Secretary of Health and Human Services to promulgate standards for a universal health identifier that will be assigned to each individual (i.e., patient), employer, health plan, and health care provider for use in the health care system. The decision to implement a universal health identifier and the particular design of the identifier have significant implications for patient privacy to the extent that they facilitate or impede the linking of records between and among institutions.[13]

The ability to link patient records among health care organizations has many advantages in the provision of care, epidemiological research, and the analysis of care and utilization patterns. For example, it is generally the case that physicians can provide better care if they have a complete patient record on which they can base clinical decisions. In some instances, insurance fraud can also be detected more easily when more complete patient records are available. The ability to link health information with other types of information such as employment, education, driving record, credit history, previous arrests and convictions, purchasing habits, telephone conversations, and e-mail exchanges, however, is more

---

[13]For example, in 1973 an advisory panel to the U.S. Department of Health, Education, and Welfare noted that, while not opposed to a universal identifier in the abstract, the members believed that, in practice, the dangers inherent in establishing such an identifier without legal and social safeguards against the abuse of electronic personal information would far outweigh any of its practical benefits. See U.S. Department of Health, Education, and Welfare. 1973. *Records, Computers, and the Rights of Citizens,* U.S. Government Printing Office, Washington, D.C. A similar conclusion was reached by a committee empaneled by the National Research Council. See National Research Council. 1972. *Databanks in a Free Society: Computers, Record Keeping, and Privacy,* National Academy of Sciences, Washington, D.C.

BOX 6.2
Possible Legislative Options for Addressing Systemic Concerns

Patients currently have few rights regarding the privacy of health information contained in private databases, beyond those provided at the state level. State laws are inconsistent, often incomplete, and difficult to prosecute. A number of initiatives could be pursued to give patients greater rights regarding the protection of health information. Should the nation wish to pursue a public policy course that places greater emphasis on the privacy and security of patient-specific health information, legislation (or, equivalently, regulation with the force of law) may be needed. The committee believes that legislation of the following types could enhance the privacy of health-related information.

• *Legislation to restrict access to patient-identifiable health information based on the intended use.* For example, legislation could define *acceptable* activities to include (1) delivery of care to patients; (2) reviews of claims for payment; (3) research uses that are approved by institutional review boards (see Chapter 5); (4) analyses of the quality of care and cost of care conducted by care providers and those at financial risk for care; and (5) the detection or prevention of fraud, such as billing for multiple prescriptions or for services that were never rendered. In this last case, such efforts should be sanctioned by the organization and subject to external audit to demonstrate their necessity, utility, and conformance to organizational practices. The legislation could define all uses of patient-identifiable information outside the prescribed set to be illegal and subject to civil and/or criminal penalties.

• *Legislation to prohibit specific practices of concern to patients.* For example, legislation could prevent self-insured employers from making individual employment decisions on the basis of patient-specific health information (as long as the

---

contentious. Economic and other forces create incentives to link individual patient data in ways that may well be detrimental to patient interests. For example, linkages of patient information with purchasing and financial information can subject individuals to marketing campaigns for new or existing therapies. Patient information linked to employment may create incentives for denying an otherwise qualified individual a job.

Recommendation 4: Any effort to develop a universal patient identifier should weigh the presumed advantages of such an identifier against potential privacy concerns. Any method used to identify patients and to link patient records in a health care environment should be evaluated against the privacy criteria listed below.

1. The method should be accompanied by an explicit policy framework that defines the nature and character of linkages that violate patient privacy and specifies legal or other sanctions for creating such linkages. That framework should derive from the national debate advocated in Recommendation 3.

employee is still able to perform his or her job functions). Legislation with this effect would eliminate much of the economic incentive for such parties to obtain patient-specific health information and thus reduce many concerns about patient privacy. Although the Americans with Disabilities Act provides some protection of this sort, it applies only to specific predefined disabilities and not to health conditions as a whole.

• *Legislation to establish information rights for patients.* As noted in Chapter 2 consumers have few legally enforceable rights regarding the privacy and security of their medical information. Today, patients have no legal basis on which to demand disclosure of information flows, access to their own health records, or redress for breaches of privacy. Passage of the Health Insurance Portability and Accountability Act is a first step toward giving patients greater ability to protect their health information, but efforts to extend the fair information practice requirements of the Privacy Act of 1974 to the private sector (including all organizations that collect, process, store, or transmit electronic health information) would empower the consumer population with enforceable rights and create a powerful force for protecting the privacy and security of sensitive information.

• *Legislation to enable a health privacy ombudsman to take legal action.* Most operating concepts of privacy ombudsmen are advisory in nature. In some instances, however, the office of privacy ombudsman has greater authority. For example, in Germany, data protection councils operate at the national level to field complaints from patients and conduct investigations as necessary.

The committee notes that legislation in all of these areas has implications that go far beyond the question of protecting the privacy interests of consumers, and realizes that making recommendations about the desirability of such legislation is beyond its expertise and charge.

2. It should facilitate the identification of parties that link records so that those who make improper linkages can be held responsible for their creation.

3. It should be unidirectional to the degree that is technically feasible: it should facilitate the appropriate linking of health records given information about the patient or provided by the patient (such as the patient's identifier), but prevent a patient's identity from being easily deduced from a set of linked health records or from the identifier iteself.

The first criterion requires that the nation decide which types of record linkages will be legal or illegal. The United States has applied this approach sporadically to protect certain types of information. For example, the perceived unfairness of using videotape rental records in the fight against the confirmation of Judge Bork for a seat on the Supreme Court led to the adoption of a law that specifically prohibits such a practice. The same law does not apply, however, to other types of records. In practice, it is difficult to legislate a prohibition on the collection of such data because institutions often have a legitimate need for the information. Prohibitions must therefore focus on the uses of such data. Unscrupulous people could, of course, still collect, collate, and use such data in ways that are prohibited, but the threat of well-defined and rigorously enforced legal sanctions would help limit such abuses.

The second criterion helps to make such a policy framework enforceable by reducing or eliminating opportunities to create improper linkages between records. If a visible and overt act is necessary to link information, illegal or unauthorized attempts to link information from various sources can be detected and traced, and guilty parties sanctioned. For example, if financial databases and health information databases used different identifiers, linkage between financial and health information would require someone to provide a translation between the different identifiers. If linkage of health and financial information without explicit patient consent were defined as a prohibited act, the fact that a linkage had been made would be an obvious indicator that a prohibited act had occurred; the party responsible for the translation would be a logical point at which to begin an investigation.

The third criterion supports patient privacy by requiring that the patient provide some information (e.g., an identifier) that can be interpreted as patient authorization for a linkage to take place. However, unidirectional linkage prevents inference of the patient's identity from just the information contained in any collection of records.

Practical application of these criteria is difficult given existing technology, but it will become more straightforward as technologies for controlling the distribution of information, such as rights management software (see Chapter 4), become more commonplace and as additional research investigates new types of identification and records-linking schemes (see Recommendation 5). In the meantime, many health care organizations have found that they can effectively link patient records within their expanding health care systems through the creation of master patient indexes. These indexes match patient records in affiliated institutions that use differing numbering systems through the use of demographic data. Although not all records or patients can be matched unambiguously, organizations that have adopted this approach report high levels of success. Linkages with organizations outside the institution can often be accomplished with information already contained in the patient record.

The three criteria given above are meant to ensure that privacy concerns are explicitly recognized in the debate over the universal patient identifier. The committee recognizes that privacy interests are only one dimension of this debate. For example, it is also important that an identifier be structured such that it does not unduly delay or prevent the provision of care, meaning that it must allow care providers to retrieve or link patient records in an emergency situation when the patient may be unable to divulge a particular identification number or may not be carrying an identification card. Other criteria must also be considered in the debate (Box 6.3).

One often-discussed universal patient identifier is the Social Security number (SSN). The committee believes that an unmodified SSN would provide little, if any, protection against attempts to link health information with other types of personal information. Although not part of its original design, the SSN is in such broad use, not only by the Social Security Administration but also by all other branches of government and many commercial enterprises, that it almost serves the function of a universal identifier today. As such, use of the SSN raises many legitimate privacy concerns.[14] On the other hand, the SSN has several attributes that make it attractive as a universal patient identifier. Among these are the fact that the SSN forms the basis of the identifier used by the Medicare program, is contained in many existing patient records held by public and private organizations, and has an existing management infrastructure for assigning numbers.[15]

Making a recommendation for or against the use of the SSN as a universal health identifier goes beyond the committee's charge and collective expertise. However, the committee notes that the use of *any* universal health identifier raises many of the same privacy issues raised by use of the SSN. The question the nation must therefore address is whether there are ways of attaining the presumed benefits of a universal patient identifier—better-informed health care, improved detection of fraud in connection with paying for health care services, and simplification of the administration of health care benefits—without jeopardizing patient privacy.[16]

Meeting Future Technological Needs

Recommendation 5: The federal government should take steps to improve information security technologies for health care applications.

---

[14]Szolovits, Peter, and Isaac Kohane. 1994. "Against Universal Health-care Identifiers," *Journal of the American Medical Informatics Association,* Vol. 1, pp. 316-319.

[15]Hammond, W. Ed. 1997. "The Use of the Social Security Number as the Basis for the National Citizen Identifier," *White Papers—The Unpredictable Certainty: Information Infrastructure Through 2000.* National Academy Press, Washington, D.C., forthcoming.

[16]For example, through the use of a system of identifiers in which individuals have a different unique identifier for each type of data collected about them or through cryptographic means, as described in Chapter 4.

BOX 6.3
Other Possible Criteria for a Universal Patient Identifier

A universal patient identifier will have to meet other criteria in addition to those designed to protect patient privacy. The following list of criteria derives from a recent report by the Institute of Medicine on the privacy of health information. The committee neither endorses nor rejects these criteria but includes them here as examples of the other considerations that will undoubtedly enter into the debate over universal patient identifiers.

1. A universal patient identifier must be able to make the transition easily from the present record-keeping environment to the future environment. This requirement has technical dimensions. If a new identifier contains more characters than the 10 used for the Medicare identifier (the Social Security number plus a single letter), software in many systems may have to be modified and data fields may have to be redefined. Further, organizations will need to know where to apply for new numbers, to verify numbers that patients give verbally, to track down uncertainties in identification, to find current mailing addresses, and to be able to trace errors and correct them.

2. A universal patient identifier must have error-control features that make entry of a wrong number unlikely. This requirement implies that errors of many kinds are detectable and possibly correctable on the basis of the digits and characters in the identifier itself. Ideally, the identifier will protect against transpositions of characters and against single, double, or multiple errors. At minimum, the error control features must be able to indicate with high confidence whether the identifier is valid.

3. A universal patient identifier should have separate identification and authentication elements. Identification implies that individuals indicate who they are; authentication allows the system to verify with a high degree of confidence that the identification offered is valid.

4. A universal patient identifier must work in any circumstance in which health care services are rendered, whether or not the situation was anticipated in the design of the system. At minimum, the identifier should pose no impediments to the prompt, efficient delivery of health care. It must work when the patient is unable to cooperate (e.g., is unconscious or does not speak the same language as the care providers), regardless of the patient's mental and physical abilities.

5. A universal patient identifier must function anywhere in the country, in any provider's facilities and settings. It should be able to link events that have occurred at multiple providers.

6. A universal patient identifier must help minimize the opportunities for crime and abuse and perhaps help to identify their perpetrators.

SOURCE: Institute of Medicine. 1994. *Health Data in the Information Age: Use, Disclosure, and Privacy,* Molla S. Donaldson and Kathleen N. Lohr (eds.). National Academy Press, Washington, D.C., pp. 165-167.

As outlined in preceding chapters of this report, patient privacy and the security of electronic health information would be greatly improved by the use of several technologies that are currently under development. The committee has identified three sets of research areas that must be pursued: (1) technologies relevant to computer security generally; (2) technologies specific to health care concerns; and (3) testbeds for a secure health care information system.

Technologies Relevant to the Computer Security Community as a Whole

Recommendation 5.1: To facilitate the exchange of technical knowledge on information security and the transfer of information security technology, the Department of Health and Human Services should establish formal liaisons with relevant government and industry working groups. Many of the technologies that could be used to better protect health information will be developed by the computer security community regardless of the needs or demands of the health care industry. Technologies for authentication, authorization, encryption, and system reliability, for instance, apply to many areas in which information security is relevant and will continue to receive attention from researchers and technologists. Biometric identifiers are the basis for approaches to very strong authentication. Public-key cryptography can be used to solve some privacy and integrity problems but requires an administrative infrastructure to be effective; thus, promotion of a public-key infrastructure would facilitate the greater use of public-key cryptography and its applications to more secure communications and data storage. Better methods to validate software packages and authenticate their sources will be needed in a computing environment based on widespread connectivity through the Internet and remotely executable programs (e.g., Java "applets") to protect against computer viruses and Trojan horse attacks. Although the Department of Health and Human Services is represented in many non-government efforts that promote health information standards, the committee believes that the health care community has not connected adequately to the information security community. For example, a consortium for developing biometric identification techniques has recently been formed but lacks representation from health-related government organizations. The health care community must be better aware of developments outside health care and must be prepared to adopt relevant solutions developed for other industries.

Technologies Specific to Health Care

Recommendation 5.2: The Department of Health and Human Services should support research in those areas listed below that are of particular importance to the health care industry, but that might not otherwise be pursued. These technologies offer greater immediate benefit to health care than to other industries for protecting privacy interests and require specific attention and funding by health-related government agencies and industry. They include the following:

- *Methods of identifying and linking patient records.* Research is needed to find ways of indexing and linking patient records in a manner that protects patient privacy. The ideal scheme would meet the three criteria for privacy outlined in Recommendation 4. It would allow patient records to be easily indexed and linked for purposes of care and other purposes determined to be legitimate, while impeding inappropriate linkages. This research should also address the extent to which a universal identifier is needed to facilitate improved care and health-related research and to simplify administration of benefits.

- *Anonymous care and pseudonyms.* Today, a patient who wishes to remain anonymous for purposes of care faces a number of serious disadvantages. For example, patients wishing to receive care anonymously must currently pay for health services in cash. More seriously, a patient wishing to be anonymous runs a serious risk when his or her medical history is on-line, although the content of that history may be critical to providing quality medical care. The use of pseudonyms or cryptographically generated aliases may mitigate this problem in the future. An alternative might be the use of narrative templates to restrict the use of names in blocks of narrative text; a record in which names occur only in a header, can be efficiently (and perhaps automatically) purged of identifying information. For patients with strong privacy concerns, smart cards containing their medical histories might present an acceptable alternative to storing data in a hospital database or larger community-wide system. Reliable techniques for linking patient records without specific patient identification may reduce the need for assigning patients unique, universal identifiers.

- *Audit tools.* Audit trails are useful as a deterrent to improper access only if there is some possibility that an improper access will in fact be recognized as such. However, the collection of audit trails routinely generates enormous amounts of data that must then be analyzed. Automated tools to analyze audit trail data would enable much more frequent examination of accesses and thus serve a more effective deterrent role. For example, intelligent screening agents could be developed that would sort through audit data and flag some records for more thorough analysis.

- *Tools for rights enforcement and management.* The primary unsolved technical problem today relates to secondary recipients of information: today's access control tools can effectively limit primary (first-person) access to data stored on-line, but they are ineffective in controlling the subsequent distribution of data. Work on electronic watermarking (or digital fingerprinting) may provide tools with which the passage of data through a network can be tracked if not prevented. Work is also under way to develop tools that provide fine-grained access control for information. Such tools limit not only the types of information that certain recipients can receive but also the types of actions recipients can take on such information, and they can be used to make audit trail entries on each access action. For example, they may prevent recipients from directly printing the information, storing it on their own computer systems, or forwarding it to another user.[17] More effective tools for rights enforcement and management would help to control secondary distribution of data.

Testbeds for Privacy and Security

Recommendation 5.3: The Department of Health and Human Services should fund experimental testbeds that explore different approaches to access control that hold promise for being inexpensive and easy to incorporate into existing operations and that allow access during emergency circumstances. Today, the trade-offs between the benefits and cost of greater access to electronic health information are not well understood, with the result that decision makers in health care organizations lack a sound analytical basis from which to determine the appropriate level of attention to protecting information. Research is needed that better explicates the costs and benefits of various levels and types of information protection so that decision makers need not function in a vacuum. The Internet Engineering Task Force has been successful in developing standards through a process of trial-and-error development of representative networked systems. Such an approach may prove useful for developing privacy and security standards in health care and may

---

[17]Of course, it is fundamentally impossible to prevent redistribution entirely. For example, nothing can prevent the recipient of data from photographing a screen and distributing the screen image. Still, making redistribution more difficult is a meaningful step to take.

be more successful than attempts to develop standards through traditional committee structures.

Similar research in the health care field could provide useful insight into effective practices and generate information that health care organizations might use to judge the efficacy, cost, and accessibility of varying approaches to privacy and security. Although the National Library of Medicine has funded the development of numerous testbeds to explore health care applications of the national information infrastructure, these efforts do not have as their primary focus attempts to explore privacy and security practices. A number of targeted security testbeds would provide useful information to the health care industry.

CONCLUDING REMARKS

The recommendations outlined in this chapter are not meant to be the final word on privacy and security in health care applications of information technology. Over time, the availability of new technology, experience with security management, changes in the structure of the health care industry, changes in the threats posed against information and communications systems, and changes in the public policy environment will require a reevaluation of effective practices. As witnessed to date, the increased capability of information technology in health care, such as electronic medical records, will continually force society to address policy issues that before could be left dormant. Yet, while the nation struggles with legislative initiatives related to privacy, the recommended practices outlined above demonstrate that meaningful steps can be taken to reduce the risk of improper disclosure at an organizational level. The committee believes that these recommendations can help to address concerns about patient information outlined in the Alice scenario in Chapter 3 and can pave the way for more productive, secure applications of information technology to health care (Box 6.4).

BOX 6.4
Charlotte's Data Flows

Charlotte, Alice and Bob's daughter, grew up in a world that refused to stand still. Charlotte was 5 when the managed care firm purchased her pediatrician's practice, and from that age, her primary medical record was kept electronically. Fueled by increasingly available and cheap computing and communications technologies, continuing attempts to control health care costs, and the need for easier access to expert specialists, telemedicine became more common. Alice frequently used her home computer to consult medical references and get additional information about Charlotte's childhood illnesses and injuries. When Charlotte was 10, the managed care firm started a program to make its patients' medical records available to them electronically. Because this was part of an initiative to attract more patients, the firm publicized the program widely and paid particular attention to ensuring that records would be released only to properly identified individuals. Alice, Bob, and Charlotte decided to join the program and were each issued a plastic card to use for authenticating requests. When Charlotte graduated from high school and went away to college, she decided to take a copy of her medical records with her. She used her card to authorize the electronic transmission of her health records to her college's student health services program.

How Did This Come About?

A number of publicized privacy violations that damaged some of their competitors had alerted senior managers of the care firm to vulnerabilities in its own procedures. In response, the firm revised its procedures to reduce the exposure of its patients' records to other groups. Samples sent to outside laboratories for analysis were encoded with numbers, rather than names, so that results could be provided anonymously. Audit trails were incorporated in the provider's own systems, and policies were established to allow patients to review the audit logs. It became straightforward to remove direct patient identification from records released to groups that did not have a legitimate need for that information. When patient-identified records were released, means were provided to "fingerprint" them with hidden information in order to detect abuses. Under the medical records protection laws that had been enacted, violations traced back through these fingerprints could be prosecuted as criminal offenses, and patients could also sue for damages. With these controls in place, management realized that it was now in a position to offer the new patient access record service without exposing itself to undue risks and that its well-developed systems could lead to a competitive edge.

How Were the Risks Reduced?

First, the communications infrastructure had been made much more resistant to eavesdropping by the incorporation of practical cryptography. Built into the communications network interface at each home was a privacy service module that incorporated a private key and could negotiate a new key for each communication session, entirely transparent to the communicating parties. These facilities had first been used to ensure the integrity and confidentiality of real-time telemedicine links and record transfers.

continued on next page

Box 6.4 Continued

As described above, the firm had upgraded its electronic record system to incorporate access controls and audit trails so that accesses by its employees could be adequately tracked, and properly authenticated prescriptions could be issued directly from the system to local pharmacies. To support the new service, a special, patient-only access system had been added that replicated records from the system used by providers but had no other access to it. In addition to being able to examine her health records, Charlotte was able to review a list of all the people who had accessed her records and the purpose of each access.

To be sure that a request for Charlotte's records came from her and not from someone else in the household, the firm also offered each of its patients a card that could be used in authenticating requests. The card avoided using the Social Security number for this purpose because those numbers were too widely available to be used for authentication. The card was used by the firm to identify its patients unambiguously, thereby reducing the paperwork required on each office visit and, in some cases, improving emergency treatment.

Bibliography

Alpert, Sheri. 1993. "CFP'93: Medical Records, Privacy, and Health Care Reform," a paper to appear as part of a larger work in progress; downloaded May 15, 1996, from www.cpsr.org.

American Bar Association. 1995. "Digital Signature Tutorial," available on-line at www.state.ut.us/ccjj/digsig/dsut-tut.htm; downloaded February 23, 1996.

American Law Institute. 1976. *Restatement (Second) of the Law of Torts*, § 652D.

American Medical Association. 1994. "Confidentiality: Computers," *Code of Medical Ethics*, American Medical Association, Chicago, Ill.

American National Standards Institute (ANSI), Healthcare Informatics Standards Planning Panel. 1992. "Charter Statement," ANSI, September.

Anderson, Ross J. 1996. "An Update on the BMA Security Policy," *Notes of the Workshop on Personal Information Security, Engineering and Ethics*, University of Cambridge, England, June 21-22.

Anderson, Ross J. 1996. *Security in Clinical Information Systems*. British Medical Association (as commissioned by the BMA Information Technology Committee), London, England, January.

Andrew, William F., and Richard S. Dick. 1995. "Applied Information Technology: A Clinical Perspective," *Computers in Nursing* 13(3):118-122.

Argyris, Chris. 1994. "Good Communication That Blocks Learning," *Harvard Business Review*, July-August, pp. 77-85.

Aries, Phillipe, and Georges Duby (eds.). 1987. *A History of Private Life*, Vols. 1-5. Belknap Press of Harvard University Press, Cambridge, Mass.

Arnold, Stephen E. 1996. "The Key to Security," *Upside*, April, pp. 78-88.

Associated Press. 1996. "Confidential AIDS Data Given to Paper," *Washington Post*, September 20, p. A7.

Auerbach, Stuart. 1997. "Two Blue Cross Plans in Area Agree to Merge," *Washington Post*, January 15, pp. C10 and C12.

197

Barrows, Randolph C., Jr., and Paul D. Clayton. 1996. "Privacy, Confidentiality, and Electronic Medical Records," *Journal of the American Medical Informatics Association* 3(2):139-148.

Bass, Alison. 1995. "Computerized Medical Data Put Privacy on the Line," *Boston Globe*, February 22, p. Metro/1.

Beth, Thomas. 1995. "Confidential Communication on the Internet," *Scientific American*, December, pp. 88-91.

Biddle, Brad. 1996. "Digital Signature Legislation: Some Reasons for Concern," available on-line at pwa.acusd.edu/~prc; downloaded February 20, 1996.

Billings, Paul, and Jon Beckwith. 1992. "Genetic Testing in the Workplace: A View from the USA," *Trends in Genetics* 8(6):198-202.

Billings, Paul R., Mel A. Kohn, Margaret de Cuevas, Jonathan Beckwith, Joseph S. Alper, and Marvin R. Natowicz. 1992. "Discrimination as a Consequence of Genetic Testing," *American Journal of Human Genetics* 50:476-482.

Biometrics in Human Services User Group Newsletter, Vol. 1, No. 1, July 1996.

Bloom, Charles. 1995. "Information Services: When Management Loses Control," *Healthcare Informatics*, June, pp. 104-108.

Bobinski, Mary Anne. 1990. "Unhealthy Federalism," *U.C. Davis Law Review* 24(255).

Bouchier, F., J.S. Ahrens, and G. Wells. 1996. "Laboratory Evaluation of the IriScan Prototype Biometric Identifier," Sandia Report SAND96-1033. Sandia National Laboratories, Albuquerque, N. Mex., April.

Brelis, Matthew. 1995. "Patients' Files Allegedly Used for Obscene Calls," *Boston Globe*, April 11, pp. 1 and 6.

Bulger, R.J. 1987. "The Search for a New Ideal," pp. 9-21 in *In Search of the Modern Hippocrates*, R.J. Bulger (ed.). University of Iowa Press, Iowa City, Iowa.

Burgdorf, Jr., Robert L. 1991. "The Americans with Disabilities Act," *Harvard C.R.-C.L. Law Review* 26(413):434-437.

Caruso, Jeff. 1996. "The Enterprise and the Net," *Interactive Age Online*, available on-line at techweb.cmp.com/ia/0219issue/0219midman.html; downloaded February 21, 1996.

Cavoukian, Ann. 1996. "Go Beyond Security—Build in Privacy: One Does Not Equal the Other," paper presented at *Cardtech/Securtech '96 Conference*, Atlanta, Ga., May 14-16.

Center for Democracy and Technology (CDT). 1996. *Privacy and Health Information Systems: A Guide to Protecting Patient Confidentiality*. CDT, Washington, D.C.

Chapman, D. Brent, and Elizabeth D. Zwicky. 1995. *Building Internet Firewalls*. O'Reilly & Associates, Inc., Sebastopol, Calif.

Chaum, David. 1992. "Achieving Electronic Privacy," *Scientific American*, August, pp. 96-101.

Cheswick, William R., and Steven M. Bellovin. 1994. *Firewalls and Internet Security*. Addison-Wesley, Reading, Mass.

Clayton, Ellen Wright, Karen K. Steinberg, Muin J. Khoury, Elizabeth Thomson, Lori Andrews, Mary Jo Ellis Kahn, Loretta M. Kopelman, and Joan O. Weiss. 1995. "Informed Consent for Genetic Research on Stored Tissue Samples," *Journal of the American Medical Association* 274(22):1786-1792.

CNN Interactive. 1996. "Yeltsin Had Heart Attack During Russian Elections," September 21, 1996, available on-line at www.cnn.com.

Cohen, Susan. 1996. "Tangled Lifeline," *Washington Post*, August 18, p. W11.

Computer-based Patient Record Institute (CPRI). 1995. *Guidelines for Establishing Information Security Policies at Organizations Using Computer-based Patient Record Systems*, CPRI Work Group on Confidentiality, Privacy, and Security. CPRI, Schaumburg, Ill., February.

Computer-based Patient Record Institute (CPRI). 1995. *Guidelines for Information Security Education Programs at Organizations Using Computer-based Patient Record Systems*, CPRI Work Group on Confidentiality, Privacy, and Security. CPRI, Schaumburg, Ill., June.

Computer-based Patient Record Institute (CPRI). 1996. *Guidelines for Managing Information Security Programs*, Work Group on Confidentiality, Privacy, and Security. CPRI, Schaumburg, Ill., January.

Computer-based Patient Record Institute (CPRI). 1996. *Sample Confidentiality Statements and Agreements for Organizations Using Computer-based Patient Record Systems*, Work Group on Confidentiality, Privacy, and Security. CPRI, Schaumburg, Ill., May.

Computer-based Patient Record Institute (CPRI). 1996. *Security Features for Computer-based Patient Record Systems*. CPRI, Schaumburg, Ill., September.

Computer Science and Telecommunications Board, National Research Council. 1991. *Computers at Risk: Safe Computing in the Information Age*. National Academy Press, Washington, D.C.

Computer Science and Telecommunications Board, National Research Council. 1996. *Cryptography's Role in Securing the Information Society*. National Academy Press, Washington, D.C.

Computer Science and Telecommunications Board, National Research Council. 1996. "Observed Practices for Improving the Security and Confidentiality of Electronic Health Information: Interim Report." National Academy Press, Washington, D.C., September.

Constance, Paul. 1996. "Multi-level Security—Not Now," *Government Computer News*, July 15, p. 60.

Consumer Reports. 1994. "Who's Reading Your Medical Records?," October, pp. 628-632.

Council on Competitiveness. 1996. *Highway to Health: Transforming U.S. Health Care in the Information Age*. Council on Competitiveness, Washington, D.C., March.

Crispell, Kenneth A., and Carlos F. Gomez. 1988. *Hidden Illness in the White House*. Duke University Press, Durham, N.C.

Dang, Dennis K., Jeffrey M. Pont, and Mitchell A. Portnoy. 1996. "Episode Treatment Groups: An Illness Classification System and Episode Building System, Part I," *Medical Interface*, March, pp. 118-122.

Daugman, J.G. 1993. "High Confidence Visual Recognition of Persons by a Test of Statistical Independence," *IEEE Transactions on Pattern Analysis and Machine Intelligence* 15(11):1148-1161.

Deloitte and Touche LLP. 1996. *U.S. Hospitals and the Future of Health Care*. Deloitte and Touche, Philadelphia.

Detmer, Don E., and Elaine B. Steen. 1993. "Patient Records in the Information Age," *Issues in Science and Technology*, Vol. 9, No. 3, pp. 24-27.

Detmer, Don E., and Elaine B. Steen. 1996. "Shoring Up Protection of Personal Health Data," *Issues in Science and Technology*, Summer, Vol. 12, No. 4, pp. 73-78.

Diffie, Whitfield. 1988. "The First Ten Years of Public-Key Cryptography," *Proceedings of the IEEE*, Vol. 76, No. 5, May, pp. 560-577.

Dunn, Ashley. 1996. "Tracking Crumbs of Data That Threaten to Define Us," *New York Times*, CyberTimes, May 12; available on-line at www.nytimes.com.

Edgar, Harold, and David J. Rothman. 1995. "The Institutional Review Board and Beyond: Future Challenges to the Ethics of Human Experimentation," *Milbank Quarterly* 73:489-506.

Elie, Benoit, and Alice Labreque. 1992. "Minimum Requirements for the Security of Computerized Records of Health and Social Services Network Clients," Commission d'acces a l'information, Province of Quebec, Canada, April.

Evans, R. Scott, Robert A. Larsen, John P. Burke, Reed M. Gardner, Frederick A. Meier, Jay A. Jacobson, Marilyn T. Conti, Julie T. Jacobson, and Russell K. Hulse. 1986. "Computer Surveillance of Hospital-Acquired Infections and Antibiotic Use," *Journal of the American Medical Association* 256(8):1007-1011.

Farkas, Charles M., and Suzy Wetlaufer. 1996. "The Ways Chief Executive Officers Lead," *Harvard Business Review,* May-June, pp. 110-122.

Ferraiolo, David, and Richard Kuhn, "Role-based Access Controls," a summary of ongoing work at the National Institute of Standards and Technology, available on-line at nemo.ncsl.nist.gov/rbac/.

Fisher, Lawrence M. 1996. "Health On-Line: A Participatory Brand of Medicine," *New York Times,* June 24.

Fisher, Lawrence M. 1996. "Netscape's Founder Begins a New Venture," *New York Times,* June 18.

Flaherty, David H. 1995. "Privacy and Data Protection in Health and Medical Information," notes for presentation to the 8th World Congress on Medical Informatics, Vancouver, B.C., Canada, July 27, available on-line at latte.cafe.net/gvc/foi/presentations/health.html; downloaded May 15, 1996.

Flynn, Laurie J. 1996. "Company Stops Providing Access to Social Security Numbers," *New York Times,* June 13; available on-line at www.nytimes.com.

Flynn, Laurie J. 1996. "Group to Monitor Web Sites for Respect of Consumer Privacy," *New York Times,* July 16; available on-line at www.nytimes.com.

Frawley, Kathleen A. 1994. "Confidentiality in the Computer Age," *RN,* July, pp. 59-60.

Freudenheim, Milt. 1996. "Blue Cross Groups Seek Profit, and States Ask Share of Riches," *New York Times,* March 25, p. A1.

Friend, Tim. 1996. "Genetic Findings Used to Deny Jobs, Coverage," *USA Today,* April 15, pp. A1 and A3.

Friend, Tim. 1996. "Researchers Uncover Genetic Discrimination," *USA Today,* August 6; available on-line at www.usatoday.com.

Fulginiti, Vincent. 1996. "The Challenge of Primary Care for Academic Health Centers," pp. 247-252 in M. Osterweis et al. (eds.), *The U.S. Health Workforce: Power, Politics and Policy.* Association of Academic Health Centers, Washington D.C.

Ganesan, Ravi, and Ravi Sandhu. 1994. "Securing Cyberspace," *Communications of the ACM,* November, pp. 29-40.

Garfinkel, Simson L. 1996. "Cryptography," paper presented at Conference on Technological Assaults on Privacy, Rochester Institute of Technology, Rochester, New York, April 18-19.

Garfinkel, Simson, and Gene Spafford. 1996. *Practical UNIX and Internet Security,* 2nd edition. O'Reilly and Associates, Inc., Cambridge, Mass.

Geller, Lisa N., Joseph S. Alper, Paul R. Billings, Carol I. Barash, Jonathan Beckwith, and Marvin R. Natowicz. 1996. "Individual, Family, and Societal Dimensions of Genetic Discrimination: A Case Study Analysis," *Science and Engineering Ethics* 2(1):71-88.

Gellman, Robert. 1984. "Prescribing Privacy: The Uncertain Role of the Physician in the Protection of Patient Privacy," *North Carolina Law Review* 62(255):274-278.

Gellman, Robert. 1996. "Individual Lookups: Crisis or Challenge to DMA's Privacy Policy?," *DM News,* April 22, p. 12.

General Accounting Office. 1996. *Information Security: Computer Attacks at Department of Defense Pose Increasing Risks.* General Accounting Office, Washington, D.C., May.

General Accounting Office. 1996. *U.S. Postal Service: Improved Oversight Needed to Protect Privacy of Address Changes.* General Accounting Office, Washington, D.C., August.

Glowniak, Jerry V., and Marilyn K. Bushway. 1994. "Computer Networks as a Medical Resource: Accessing and Using the Internet," *Journal of the American Medical Association* 271(24):1934-1939.

Gobis, Linda J. 1994. "Computerized Patient Records: Start Preparing Now," *Journal of Nursing Administration* 24(9):15-16.

Gobis, Linda J. 1995. "Bedside Computers and Confidentiality," *American Journal of Nursing*, October, pp. 75-76.

Goldman, Janlori. 1995. "Statement Before the Senate Committee on Labor and Human Resources on S.1360, the Medical Records Confidentiality Act of 1995," November 14. [also letter dated April 29, 1996, to Senators Kassebaum and Kennedy and *CDT Policy Post*, Vols. 2(11) and 2(14).]

Golob, Randy. 1994. "America's Best Networked Healthcare Organizations," *Healthcare Informatics*, November, pp. 84-88.

Gordon & Glickson. 1995. *Overcoming the Legal Challenges in Converting to a Computerized Medical Record*. Gordon & Glickson, Chicago, Ill.; available on-line at www.ggtech.com.

Gordon & Glickson. 1995. *Second Annual Computer-based Patient Records Survey*. Gordon & Glickson, Chicago, Ill.; available on-line at www.ggtech.com.

Gordon & Glickson. 1996. *A Model Defining and Exploring Information Transactions Between Public Health and Healthcare Organizations: Legal and Data Security Issues*. Gordon & Glickson, Chicago, Ill.; available on-line at www.ggtech.com.

Gorman, Christine. 1996. "Big Brother Wants You Healthy," *TIME Magazine*, May 6, p. 62.

Gorman, Christine. 1996. "Who's Looking at Your Files?," *TIME Magazine*, May 6, pp. 60-62.

Gostin, Lawrence O., and Zita Lazzarini. 1995. "Childhood Immunization Registries: A National Review of Public Health Information Systems and the Protection of Privacy," *Journal of the American Medical Association* 274(22):1793-1799.

Gostin, Lawrence O., Zita Lazzarini, Verla S. Neslund, and Michael T. Osterholm. 1996. "The Public Health Information Infrastructure: A National Review of the Law on Health Information Privacy," *Journal of the American Medical Association* 275(24):1921-1927.

Graubart, Richard D. 1995. *Securing a Healthcare Information System*. The MITRE Corporation, Bedford, Mass., June.

Greenberg, Daniel S. 1996. "Nemesis of Privacy," *Washington Post*, August 1, p. A23.

Grigsby, Jim, Robert E. Schlenker, Margaret M. Kaehny, Elliot J. Sandberg, Phoebe Lindsey Barton, Peter W. Shaughnessy, Andrew M. Kramer, and Susan K. Beale. 1994. "Analysis of Expansion of Access to Care Through Use of Telemedicine," paper downloaded June 19, 1995, from gopher://gopher.hpcc.gov.

Gritzalis, D., I. Kantzavelou, S. Katsikas, and A. Patel. 1995. "A Classification of Health Information System Security Flaws," pp. 453-463 in *Proceedings of the 11th International Information Security Conference (IFIP SEC '95)*, J. Eloff and S.H. von Solms (eds.). Chapman & Hall, South Africa.

Gruley, Bryan, and Thomas M. Burton. 1996. "Drugstores Request Changes in Lilly's Acquisition of PCS," *Wall Street Journal*, August 1, available on-line at www.wsj.com.

Hafferty, Frederic, and Donald Light. 1995. "Professional Dynamics and the Changing Nature of Medical Work," *Journal of Health and Social Behavior*, extra issue, pp. 132-153.

Hall, Eric. 1996. "Interactive Network Design Manual: Internet Firewall Essentials," *Network Computing*, April 22, available on-line at techweb.cmp.com/nc/netdesign/wall1.html.

Hammond, W. Ed. 1992. "Security, Privacy, and Confidentiality: A Perspective," *Journal of Health Information Management Research* 1(2):1-8.

Hammond, W. Ed. 1997. "The Use of the Social Security Number as the Basis for the National Citizen Identifier," *White Papers—the Unpredictable Certainty: Information Infrastructure Through 2000*. National Academy Press, Washington, D.C., forthcoming.

Healthcare Information and Management Systems Society (HIMSS). 1995. "Appendix IV: JCAHO Information Management Standards," *1995 HIMSS Proceedings*. HIMSS, Chicago, Ill.

Health Data Network News. 1996. "Houston Docs On Call Will Use the Internet to Get Patient Records," June 20, pp. 1 and 8.

Health Data Network News. 1996. "Claims Over the Internet? It's Happening," May 20, p. 1.

Health Data Network News. 1996. "The Pharmacy Fund Looks for Rapid Expansion of Its Rapid RxEmit Program," January 20, p. 5.

Health Insurance Association of America. 1996. *Source Book of Health Insurance Data*. Health Insurance Association of America, Washington, D.C.

Health Management Technology. 1995. "I/T Sales to Soar Next Five Years," December, p. 10.

Holbrook, P., and J. Reynolds (eds.). 1991. "Site Security Handbook," IETF RFC 1244, July, available on-line at www.ietf.org.

Holmes, J.P., L.J. Wright, and R.L. Maxwell. 1991. "A Performance Evaluation of Biometric Identification Devices," Sandia Report SAND91-0276. Sandia National Laboratories, Albuquerque, N. Mex., June.

Information and Privacy Commissioner (Ontario, Canada) and Registratiekamer (The Netherlands). 1995. *Privacy-Enhancing Technologies: The Path to Anonymity*. Volume I, [no publisher/location noted], August.

Information Highway Advisory Council. 1996. *Building the Information Society: Moving Canada into the 21st Century*, Catalog No. C2-302/1996. Minister of Supply and Services Canada, Ottawa, Ontario.

Information Infrastructure Task Force (IITF). 1995. "Privacy and the National Information Infrastructure: Principles for Providing and Using Personal Information," Privacy Working Group, Information Policy Committee, IITF, final version dated June 6; downloaded May 9, 1996, from www.iitf.doc.gov.

Information Week. 1996. Vol. 3 (June), p. 12.

Inside Healthcare Computing. 1996. "How a 13-Year-Old Breached HIS Security, Made Phony AIDS Calls," 6(8), March 4, pp. 1-2.

Institute of Medicine. 1991. *The Computer-based Patient Record: An Essential Technology for Health Care*, Richard S. Dick and Elaine B. Steen, eds. National Academy Press, Washington, D.C.

Institute of Medicine. 1994. *Health Data in the Information Age: Use, Disclosure, and Privacy*, Molla S. Donaldson and Kathleen N. Lohr (eds.). National Academy Press, Washington, D.C.

Institute of Medicine. 1994. "Regional Health Databases, Health Services Research, and Confidentiality," a summary paper of a workshop, National Implications of the Development of Regional Health Database Organizations, January 31- February 1, Washington, D.C.

Institute of Medicine. 1995. *Real People, Real Problems: An Evaluation of the Long-term Care Ombudsman Programs of the Older Americans Act*, National Academy Press, Washington, D.C.

Jeffrey, Nancy Ann. 1996. "Getting Access to Your Medical Records May Be Limited, Costly—or Impossible," *Wall Street Journal*, July 31, pp. C1 and C21.

Jeffrey, Nancy Ann. 1996. "'Wellness Plans' Try to Target Those Who Aren't So Well," *Wall Street Journal*, June 20; available on-line at www.wsj.com.

Kaluzny, Arnold D., Howard S. Zuckerman, and Thomas C. Ricketts III (eds.). 1995. *Part-ners for the Dance: Forming Strategic Alliances in Health Care.* Health Administration Press, Ann Arbor, Mich.

Kanter, Rosabeth Moss, David V. Summers, and Barry A. Stein. 1986. "The Future of Workplace Alternatives," *Management Review* 75(7):30-33.

Kanter, Rosabeth Moss. 1994. "Collaborative Advantage: The Art of Alliances," *Harvard Business Review,* July-August, pp. 96-108

Keeton, W. Page (ed.) 1984. *Prosser and Keeton on the Law of Torts.* West Publishing Company, St. Paul, Minn.

Kemmerer, Richard A. 1994. "Security, Computer," *Encyclopedia of Software Engineering.* John Wiley & Sons Inc., New York, pp. 1153-1164.

Khanna, Raman (ed.). 1993. *Distributed Computing: Implementation and Management Strategies.* Prentice-Hall, Englewood Cliffs, N.J.

Knecht, Bruce. 1996. "Click! Doctor to Post Patient Files on Net," *Wall Street Journal,* February 20, p. B1.

Kohane, Isaac S., F.J. van Wingerde, James C. Fackler, Christopher Cimino, Peter Kilbridge, Shawn Murphy, Henry Chueh, David Rind, Charles Safran, Octo Barnett, and Peter Szolovits. 1996. "Sharing Electronic Medical Records Across Multiple Heterogeneous and Competing Institutions," available on-line at www.emrs.org/publications/.

Kohl, J., and C. Neuman. 1993. "The Kerberos Network Authentication Service (V5)," RFC 1510, Internet Working Group, available on-line at ds.internic.net/rfc/rfc1510.txt.

Korpman, Ralph A., and Thomas L. Lincoln. 1988. "The Computer-Stored Medical Record," *Journal of the American Medical Association* 259(23):3454-3456.

Laban, James. 1996. *Privacy Issues Surrounding Personal Identification Systems,* available on-line at www.dss.state.ct.us/digital.htm.

Larkin, T.J., and Sandar Larkin. 1996. "Reaching and Changing Frontline Employees," *Harvard Business Review,* May-June, pp. 95-104.

Lawrence, Larry M. 1994. "Safeguarding the Confidentiality of Automated Medical Information," *Journal on Quality Improvement* 20(11):639-646.

Lee, Therese. 1996. "Medicine Prof Testifies in DNA Case," *Stanford Daily,* April 24, pp. 1-2.

Lewin, Tamar. 1996. "Questions of Privacy Roil Arena of Psychotherapy," *New York Times,* May 22; available on-line at www.nytimes.com.

Lincoln, Thomas L. 1994. "Traveling the New Information Highway," *Journal of the American Medical Association* 271(24):1955-1956.

Linowes, David F. 1989. *Privacy in America: Is Your Private Life in the Public Eye?* University of Illinois Press, Urbana, Ill., p. 42.

Linowes, David. 1996. "A Research Survey of Privacy in the Workplace," an unpublished white paper available from the University of Illinois at Urbana-Champaign.

Louis Harris and Associates (in association with Alan Westin). 1993. *Health Information Privacy Survey 1993.* A survey conducted for EQUIFAX Inc. by Louis Harris and Associates, New York.

Louis Harris and Associates. 1995. *Equifax-Harris Mid-Decade Consumer Privacy Survey,* Study No. 953012. Louis Harris and Associates, New York.

Marbach, William D. 1983. "Beware: Hackers at Play," *Newsweek,* September 5, p. 42-46.

Markoff, John. 1996. "Balancing Privacy and Official Eavesdropping," *New York Times,* July 13; available on-line at www.nytimes.com.

McDonald, Clement J., and William M. Tierney. 1988. "Computer-Stored Medical Records: Their Future Role in Medical Practice," *Journal of the American Medical Association* 259(23):3433-3440.

McMenamin, Brigid. 1996. "It Can't Happen Here," *Forbes,* May 20, pp. 252-254.

McMullen, William L. 1994. *Overview of a Healthcare Information System Architecture Beyond the Computer-based Patient Record.* The MITRE Corporation, McLean, Va.

Medical Information Bureau. 1995. *Medical Information Bureau: A Consumer's Guide.* Medical Information Bureau, Westwood, Mass., September.

Medical Interface. 1996. "Drug Companies Using More Pharmacoeconomic Data in Marketing," March, pp. 38-39.

Milholland, D. Kathy, and Barbara R. Heller. 1992. "Computer-based Patient Record: From Pipe Dream to Reality," *Computers in Nursing* 10(5):191-192.

Milholland, D. Kathy. 1994. "Privacy and Confidentiality of Patient Information: Challenges for Nursing," *Journal of Nursing Adminstration* 24(2):19-24.

Miller, Benjamin. 1994. "Vital Signs of Identity," *IEEE Spectrum,* February, pp. 22-30.

Miller, Dale. 1994. "Confidentiality Safeguards for Quality Assurance Systems," *Infocare: Special Supplement to Healthcare Informatics,* April, pp. 58-62.

Miller, Frances H., and Philip A. Huvos. 1994. "Genetic Blueprints, Employer Cost-Cutting, and the Americans with Disabilities Act," *Administrative Law Review* 46(369):383.

Miller, Robert H. 1996. "Health System Integration: A Means to an End," *Health Affairs* 15(2):92-106.

Miller, S., C. Neuman, J. Schiller, and J. Saltzer. 1987. "Section E.2.1: Kerberos Authentication and Authorization System," *MIT Project Athena,* Cambridge, Mass.

Modern Healthcare. 1996. "Did You Hear the One About . . . ?," April 8, p. 52.

Molander, Roger C., Andrew S. Riddile, and Peter A. Wilson. 1996. *Strategic Information Warfare: A New Face of War,* RAND Report MR-601. RAND Corporation, Santa Monica, Calif.

Morrissey, John. 1996. "A Broader Vision: CIOs Shift Strategy to Look Beyond the Hospital," *Modern Healthcare,* March 4, pp. 110-113.

Morrissey, John. 1996. "Clinical Systems Add Market Momentum," *Modern Healthcare,* March 4, pp. 114-120, 132.

Morrissey, John. 1996. "Data Security," *Modern Healthcare,* September 30, pp. 32-40.

Morrissey, John. 1996. "Full Speed Ahead," *Modern Healthcare,* March 4, pp. 97-108.

Munro, Neil. 1996. "Infotech Reshapes Health Care Marketplace," *Washington Technology,* August 8.

Murray, William Hugh. 1996. "Remarks of William Hugh Murray to the Committee on Health Privacy of the NRC," Deloitte & Touche LLP, Wilton, Conn., February 27.

Murrey, Katherine, Lawrence Gottlieb, and Stephen Schoenbaum. 1992. "Implementing Clinical Guidelines: A Quality Mangement Approach to Reminder Systems," *Quality Review Bulletin,* December, pp. 423-433.

National Institute of Standards and Technology. 1994. *Putting the Information Infrastructure to Work: Report of the Information Infrastructure Task Force Committee on Applications and Technology,* NIST Special Publication 857. U.S. Government Printing Office, Washington, D.C., May.

National Library of Medicine. 1996. *Current Bibliographies in Medicine: Confidentiality of Electronic Health Data,* No. 95-10. National Library of Medicine, Rockville, Md.

National Research Council. 1972. *Databanks in a Free Society: Computers, Record Keeping, and Privacy.* National Academy of Sciences, Washington, D.C.

Navarro, Robert P. 1996. "User Applications of Health Economic Data," *Medical Interface,* March, pp. 81-82.

Needham, R., and M. Schroeder. 1978. "Using Encryption for Authentication in Large Networks of Computers," *Communications of the ACM,* Vol. 21, No. 12.

Neumann, Peter. 1995. *Computer Related Risks.* Addison-Wesley, Reading, Mass.

Nichols, Nancy A. 1994. "Medicine, Management, and Mergers: An Interview with Merck's P. Roy Vagelos," *Harvard Business Review,* November-December, pp. 105-114.

Nissenbaum, Helen. 1996. "Violating Privacy in Public: Meeting the Challenges of Information Technology," draft paper presented at Conference on Technological Assaults on Privacy, Rochester Institute of Technology, Rochester, New York, April 18-19.

Office of Technology Assessment . 1993. *Protecting Privacy in Computerized Medical Information*, OTA-TCT-576. U.S. Government Printing Office, Washington, D.C.

Office of Technology Assessment. 1995. *Bringing Health Care Online: The Role of Information Technologies*. U.S. Government Printing Office, Washington, D.C.

Ornstein, Steven M., Edward Schaeffer, Ruth G. Jenkins, and Robert L. Edsall. 1996. "A Vendor Survey of Computerized Patient Record Systems," *Family Practice Management*, February, pp. 35-49.

Panettieri, Joseph C. 1995. "Ernst & Young Security Survey," *Information Week*; downloaded August 22, 1995, from www.techweb.com.

Patient Confidentiality and Privacy Work Group, Massachusetts Health Data Consortium Inc. 1996. "Confidentiality of Health Data—An Exploration of Principles, Policies, and Practices," draft paper dated March 28, presented at a public meeting in Boston sponsored by Massachusetts Health Data Consortium, Waltham, Mass.

Pharmaceutical Research and Manufacturers Association. 1996. *Industry Profile*. Pharmaceutical Research and Manufacturers Association, Washington, D.C.

Pollard, Michael R., and Hugh H. Tilson, Jr. 1996. "Implications for Managed Care Organizations of the Merck and Medco Consent," *Medical Interface*, March, pp. 60-62.

Power, Richard. 1996. "1996 CSI/FBI Computer Crime and Security Survey," *Computer Security Issues & Trends*, Vol. II, No. 2., Spring, p. 2.

PRNewswire. 1996. "Minnesota Takes the Lead on Agreement to Protect 41 Million Americans," October 25; available on-line at www.epic.org/privacy/medical/merck.txt.

Privacy Protection Study Commission. 1977. *Personal Privacy in an Information Society*. Privacy Protection Study Commission, Washington, D.C., July, Chapter 7, pp. 277-317.

Public Health Data Policy Coordinating Committee. 1995. *Making a Powerful Connection: The Health of the Public and the National Information Infrastructure*. U.S. Public Health Service, Washington, D.C.; downloaded from www.nlm.nih.gov on November 14, 1995.

Reich, Paul. 1996. "Today's Drug Utilization Review," *Medical Interface*, March, p. 12.

Riley, John. 1996. "Know and Tell: Sharing Medical Data Becomes Prescription for Profit," *Newsday*, April 2, pp. A17, A50-A51.

Riley, John. 1996. "Open Secrets: Changes in Technology, Health Insurance Making Privacy a Thing of the Past," *Newsday*, March 31, pp. A5, A41-A42.

Riley, John. 1996. "'Virtual Records': Patient Data at Click of Mouse," *Newsday*, March 31, pp. A5 and A40.

Riley, John. 1996. "When You Can't Keep a Secret: Insurers' Cost-cutters Demand Your Medical Details," *Newsday*, April 1, pp. A7, A36-A38.

Riley, John. 1996. "Will Bill Cure Ills?: Legislation on Access to Medical Data Sparks Debate," *Newsday*, April 3, pp. A19 and A53.

Rodriguez, Karen. 1996. "Pushing the Envelope," *Communications Week*, May 13, p. 37.

Rogers, L., and D. Leppard. 1995. "For Sale: Your Secret Medical Records for £150," *London Sunday Times*, November 26, pp. 1-2.

Rosnow, Ralph L., Mary Jane Rotheram-Borus, Stephen J. Ceci, Peter D. Blanck, and Gerald P. Koocher. 1993. "The Institutional Review as a Mirror of Scientific and Ethical Standards," *American Psychologist* 48(7):821-826.

Rotenberg, Marc. 1995. "Principles for Federal Privacy Protection of Medical Records," *EPIC Alert*, Vol. 2, No. 13, October 13.

Rotenberg, Marc. 1994. "Privacy and Security for Medical Information Systems," an outline of keynote address given at AHIMA conference, Seizing the Opportunity: The Power of Health Information, Las Vegas, Nevada, October.

Rothenberg, Karen. 1995. "Genetic Information and Health Insurance: State Legislative Approaches," *Journal of Law, Medicine, and Ethics* 23(312):312-319.

Rothfeder, Jeffrey. 1992. *Privacy for Sale: How Computerization Has Made Everyone's Life an Open Secret.* Simon and Schuster, New York.

Rothstein, Mark A. 1992. "Genetic Discrimination in Employment and the Americans with Disabilities Act," *Houston Law Review* 29(23):80-81.

Sack, Kevin. 1995. "House Panel to Draft Bill on AIDS Tests of Newborns," *New York Times,* July 14, p. A15.

San Francisco Chronicle. 1996. "Genetic Testing Raises Questions of Discrimination," April 15.

Schiller, Jeffrey I. 1994. "Secure Distributed Computing," *Scientific American* 271(5):72-76.

Schoeman, Ferdinand David (ed.). 1984. *Philosophical Dimensions of Privacy: An Anthology.* Cambridge University Press, Cambridge, England.

Schultz, Ellen E. 1991. "If You Use Firm's Counselors, Remember Your Secrets Could Be Used Against You," *Wall Street Journal,* May 26, pp. C1 and C6.

Schultz, Ellen E. 1994. "Open Secrets: Medical Data Gathered by Firms Can Prove Less Than Confidential," *Wall Street Journal,* May 18, p. A1.

Schwartz, John. 1996. "Insurer's Refusal to Disclose Deadly Diagnosis Leads to Legal Battle," *Washington Post,* August 4, p. A3.

Schwartz, Paul M. 1995. "European Data Protection Law and Restrictions on International Data Flows," *Iowa Law Review* 80(3): 471-496.

Schwartz, Paul M. 1995. "The Protection of Privacy in Health Care Reform," *Vanderbilt Law Review* 48(2):296-347.

Schwartz, Paul M., and Joel R. Reidenberg. 1996. *Data Privacy Law: A Study of United States Data Protection.* Michie Law Publishers, Charlottesville, Va.

Scism, Leslie. 1996. "U.S. Healthcare Antitrust Fight: Does Firm Coerce Pharmacies?," *Wall Street Journal,* May 20; available on-line at www.wsj.com.

Simpson, Roy L. 1994. "Ensuring Patient Data, Privacy, Confidentiality, and Security," *Nursing Management* 25(7):18-20.

Smith, H. Jeff. 1993. "Privacy Policies and Practices: Inside the Organizational Maze," *Communications of the ACM* 36:105-122.

Smith, H. Jeff. 1994. *Managing Privacy: Information Technology and Corporate America.* University of North Carolina Press, Chapel Hill, N.C.

Smith, H. Jeff, and Ernest A. Kallman. 1992. "Privacy Attitudes and Practices: An Empirical Study of Medical Record Directors' Perceptions," *Journal of Health Information Management Research* 1(2):9-31.

Soumerai, S., and J. Avorn. 1990. "Principles of Educational Outreach to Improve Clinical Decision Making," *Journal of the American Medical Association* 262:549-556.

Stix, Gary. 1994. "Dr. Big Brother," *Scientific American* 270(2):108-109.

Szolovits, Peter, and Isaac Kohane. 1994. "Against Universal Health-care Identifiers," *Journal of the American Medical Informatics Association* 1:316-319.

Tippit, Sarah. 1996. "A New Danger in the Age of AIDS," *Washington Post,* October 14, p. A4.

Turkington, Richard C. 1996. "Privacy and Autonomy in Cyberspace," draft discussion document presented at Conference on Technological Assaults on Privacy, Rochester Institute of Technology, Rochester, New York, April 18-19.

U.S. Department of Commerce, National Bureau of Standards. 1977. "Data Encryption Standard," *FIPS Publication 46.* National Bureau of Standards, Washington, D.C.

U.S. Department of Health, Education, and Welfare. 1973. *Records, Computers, and the Rights of Citizens*. U.S. Government Printing Office, Washington, D.C.

U.S. Department of Health and Human Services, Agency for Health Care Policy and Research. 1995. *Using Clinical Practice Guidelines to Evaluate Quality of Care*, Volume 1. U.S. Government Printing Office, Washington, D.C., March.

Vanselow, Neal. 1996. "New Health Workforce Responsibilities and Dilemmas," pages 231-242 in M. Osterweis et al. (eds.), *The U.S. Health Workforce: Power, Politics and Policy*. Association of Academic Health Centers, Washington D.C.

Venema, Wietse. 1992. "TCP WRAPPER: Network Monitoring, Access Control and Booby Traps," pp. 85-92 in *Proceedings of the Third Usenix UNIX Security Symposium*, Baltimore, Md., September.

Violino, Bob. 1996. "Internet Security: Your Worst Nightmare," *Information Week Online*, available on-line at techweb.cmp.com/iw/567/67mtsec.htm.

Violino, Bob. 1996. "The Security Facade: Are Organizations Doing Enough to Protect Themselves? This Year's IW/Ernst & Young Survey Will Shock You," *Information Week*, October 21.

Walker, John M. 1993. "Employee Retirement Income Security Act of 1974: An Overview of ERISA Pre-Emption," *American Journal of Trial Advocacy* 17(529), Fall.

Walker, Robert. 1995. "'Smart Cards' to Cut Health Costs," *Calgary Herald*, June 15; available on-line at www.southam.com/edmontonjournal/archives.

Weiss, Rick. 1996. "Hospital Reviews Criticized: Watchdog Group Says System Is Flawed," *Washington Post*, July 11, p. A23.

Whittemore, Jr., Ken. 1995. "Electronic Prescription Transmission," *National Association of Retail Druggists*, April, pp. 18-22.

Wiederhold, Gio, Michel Bilello, Vatsala Sarathy, and XioaLei Qian. 1996. "A Security Mediator for Health Care Information," *Proceedings of the 1996 AMIA Conference*, Washington, D.C., October, pp. 120-124.

Williams, Tennessee. 1947. *A Streetcar Named Desire*. New Directions, New York.

Appendixes

APPENDIX
A

Study Committee's Site Visit Guide

GENERAL PROTOCOL FOR SITE VISITS

STEP 1: Develop general field visit guide for use by all teams at all sites
- list topics to cover (see list I below)
- list questions to ask (see, "Possible Questions for Site Visit Interviews" below)
- select sites

STEP 2: Pre-visit contact
- make arrangements for visit (time, place, hotels)
- ask for documents on study issues ahead of time (see list II below)
- identify people to interview on site (see list III below)

STEP 3: Team preparation (conference calls)
- teams review documents, match to questions, identify gaps/areas in need of on-site questioning
- make final decisions regarding individuals to interview on-site

STEP 4: Generate customized site visit protocol

STEP 5: Conduct site visit
- kick off introductory meeting with CEO/CIO and all actors
- follow up with one-on-one interviews

STEP 6: Debrief/draft report
- each site visitor reports on interviews
- each site visitor summarizes his or her "picture"
- team leader assimilates inputs and drafts overall report

SITE VISIT INFORMATION

I. Topics to cover
  - Privacy policies
  - Implementation of privacy policies
  - Responsibilities for developing and enforcing policies
  - Training of employees
  - Past security incidents/events
  - Definitions of privacy, confidentiality, and security
  - Content of electronic medical records
  - Description of information system(s)
  - Perception of internal security threats
  - Perception of external security threats
  - Description of security mechanisms
  - Evaluation of security mechanisms
  - Disaster planning
  - Security/damage control plans

II. Documents/information to request ahead of time
  - Organization's mission statement
  - Organizational chart
  - Privacy and security policies
  - Enabling/implementation documents for privacy/security policies
  - Description of personnel practices for punishing violators
  - Policies on record-keeping
  - Policy for release of information from medical records
  - Information system description(s)
  - Strategic plan for information system
  - Description of security systems for information system
  - List of responsibilities within information systems department
    - who is responsible for data release internally and externally?
    - who has administrative oversight for making sure information policies are actually implemented?

III. People to interview
  - CEO (or other high-level person responsible for deciding to develop privacy policy)

- CIO
- Technical systems administrator
- Network manager
- Security director
- Medical records director
- User groups (physicians, nurses, others?)
- Legal department or counsel

POSSIBLE QUESTIONS FOR SITE VISIT INTERVIEWS

I. Organization and confidentiality policies

A1) What is the general structure of the organization? A2) What are the goals of the organization? A3) What types of services do you offer and in what types of settings? A4) To what extent do you work with affiliated health care providers?

B1) What are the organization's existing policies regarding security and confidentiality of medical records? B2) How are they stated and promulgated? B3) What information do they try to protect? B4) Are there policies targeted specifically toward electronic medical records? B5) If so, how are they different from polices directed toward paper records? B6) What balance do the policies strike between patient confidentiality and provider access?

C1) Are patients given access to their own records? If so, can they see the entire record or just an abstract? C2) Are they allowed to make corrections to their own records?

D1) Who else can information be released to (insurers, researchers, other doctors, etc.)? D2) What limits are placed on such releases? D3) Is all information released, or just some? D4) Are additional restrictions placed on "sensitive data" such as HIV tests, drug and alcohol abuse? D5) What procedures must requesters follow in order to access medical information? D6) Must patients consent to releases of medical information?

E1) What is the process by which privacy and security policies are developed and implemented? E2) Is there a committee that regularly reviews confidentiality policies? E3) Who reviewed and signed off on the existing policies? E4) Have clients/consumers been involved in the development of the confidentiality policies? E5) Have you received comments or questions from consumers regarding the information system and confidentiality or security of their data?

F1) What factors motivate and shape the development of confidentiality policies: state and federal legislation, law suits, unauthorized releases of medical information? F2) What types of liabilities do the policies protect against? F3) Do they create other liabilities/legal problems? F4)

Do policies themselves leave the organization open to suit (e.g., unfair termination or negligence)?

G1) How are violators punished? G2) How are they caught? G3) Are mechanisms in place to monitor and catch violations?

H1) What has been the response to the policy, both internally and externally? H2) What is management's view of privacy and confidentiality? H3) Who are the stakeholders in the medical information systems they use? H4) What does "security" mean to these stakeholders? H5) What information is viewed as being especially sensitive?

I1) What do you see as the primary needs for privacy and security in health care information systems? I2) How do these differ across users: providers, patients, third-party payer/insurers, public health organizations, law enforcement, researchers.

II. Data exchanges

A1) With what other institutions are data exchanged? Insurers? Government agencies (state and federal)? Other hospitals? Regulatory authorities? A2) How much of the data is exchanged? A3) Who decides on policy for what gets shared with whom? A4) What quality control mechanisms exist to ensure that policy is carried out?

III. Aggregated data

A1) What procedures are in place to handle requests for aggregate data? A2) Do researchers have access to the repository of clinical data for large-scale queries? A3) Is such access routinely available or does it have to be arranged, e.g., by ad hoc dump of data files from the operational system?

B1) If data are made available for research studies, is there any attempt to "scrub" (remove identifying information from) the data? B2) If yes, what standards are established for the degree of scrubbing, who sets such standards, and how are they verified?

C1) Is institutional review board approval required for all such studies?

D1) If a researcher is a participant in multi-institutional trials, is there hospital policy on whether shared data may retain or must have removed all identifiers?

IV. Policy implementation

A1) How/how well do specific policies actually work in practice? A2) What issues still need to be addressed? A3) Who is responsible for system security?

B1) Who is responsible for implementing privacy and security policies? B2) Is there a security officer? B3) How big is the security staff? B4)

Is responsibility centralized or distributed among a number of people? B5) If there is a central person, how is responsibility delegated to other units/people?

C1) Is there a variance between the policies for paper records and electronic records regarding security and access? C2) Are there differences in accountability for paper and electronic records?

V. Violations/problems/experiences

A1) What types of violations/incidents have occurred in the past? A2) How were they detected? By whom? A3) How were they punished? A4) Was the punishment public? A5) Who handled the punishment?

B1) Are there reporting mechanisms for apparent anomalous behavior of system or users?

C1) If violations or security breaches have occurred, how were policies, training, or systems redesigned to help prevent subsequent occurrences? C2) What resources were used?

VI. Training/education

A1) How are workers educated regarding policies? A2) Is there a system of formal training? A3) If so, who performs the training? A4) Does it include training in ethics?

B1) Do workers receive additional training as their jobs/responsibilities change? B2) Do they receive additional training/education when new facilities are added to the system or when policies change? B3) Are there refresher courses? If so, how often?

VII. Information system(s)

A1) What types of information systems are in place for storing, retrieving, and manipulating medical information? (Include satellite systems as for report writing, research.) A2) What kinds of information processing do these systems support: databases, remote access, email, web sites, other? A3) What information is on-line and not on-line?

B1) How is the system organized? It is a centralized or distributed system? B2) What is the perimeter of the system? B3) What components are considered internal to the system and which are external to it? B4) How many entry points are there in the system?

C1) What media are used to provide access from inside and outside the institution? Dial up lines? Fixed/private lines? Private networks? Public networks? C2) What is the logical and physical configuration of the communications systems

D1) Is access to the information system from outside the organization possible? D2) Is such access restricted to organization employees or is it also available to "outsiders"?

E1) What parts of the information system were supplied by vendors, and which are "home grown"?

VIII. Electronic medical record

A1) What components exist as part of the electronic medical record: problem list, medications, lab results, visit history, patient-provider relationships, bedside (clinical) measurements, full-text clinical notes, images, demographic information, including employer, financial, insurance, next of kin?

B1) Are medical records kept under a master patient identifier? B2) If not, what combination of attributes is used to identify patients? B3) If so, is the master key the SSN? B4) If the SSN is not used as the primary identifier, is it nevertheless commonly available in the medical record?

C1) How is ownership of the information contained in the record determined and managed? C2) Who is responsible for ensuring the integrity and quality of information in the patient record?

D1) What technical and non-technical means are used to ensure the integrity of data in the electronic medical record? D2) Are digital signatures or time stamps used?

E1) What types of uses are made of the electronic patient record? E2) How does medical information flow through the organization for 1) routine medical purposes (e.g., emergency room visits, outpatient visits, inpatient stays); and 2) non-routine visits (e.g., special treatment of data for particular classes of individuals, such as celebrities or criminals)?

F1) How do you respond to unusual requests for information: research projects, subpoenas, etc.? F2) How do you handle requests arriving via telephone?

IX. Security threats

A1) What do you perceive to be the threats to the system, both internal and external? A2) Are current users aware of the potential threats?

B1) What internal and external threats is your system designed to protect against? B2) Did you perform a formal threat analysis?

C1) What are the vulnerabilities of the current system? C2) What threats have not been adequately addressed? C3) What types of problems have you experienced to date—hackers, system crashes, etc.?

D1) What types of security threats have arisen to date? D2) How well does/did the system handle these threats? D3) What has been learned from such experiences?

X. Security measures
A. General Issues
1a) What general types of physical security and security technol-

ogy are used in the system: Kerberos, encryption, private lines, firewalls? 1b) To what extent does cost effectiveness affect decisions regarding security? 1c) What types of tradeoffs must be made between security capability and cost?

2a) Is a single, integrated security solution feasible? 2b) Can vendor products meet local needs, or must systems be tailored for different circumstances? 2c) Are standards available for security systems?

3a) What are 5 areas in which your organization is doing a great job regarding privacy and security?

B. Authentication

1a) What mechanisms are used for individual authentication for access? 1b) Do you have unique login for individual users? If so, what type of key is used? 1c) Who issues the key? 1d) How frequently is the key changed?

2a) How do you verify new users? 2b) How do you terminate access for employees or former employees no longer allowed into the system?

3a) Do you use passwords for authentication? 3b) What types of passwords are used? 3c) Are they selected by users or generated for them? 3d) How frequently are passwords changed? 3e) Are there limitations imposed on the types of passwords users may select?

4a) In practice are passwords routinely shared or posted? 4b) Are methods used to protect against password sharing?

5a) Are mechanisms other than keys and passwords used for authentication, such as smart cards, palm readers, voice recognition systems, address filtering gateways?

6a) Do you have an authentication server? 6b) Is information stored in encrypted form on the server?

7a) Does the information system automatically maintain audit trails of who accessed what information? 7b) What types of audit capabilities are in place? 7c) Who reviews such audit trails, and how frequently? 7d) What fraction of accesses is reviewed, and how thoroughly? 7e) Who determines review policy? 7f) What consequences are there for infractions of policy?

C. Access

1a) Is access to medical records granted to everyone, or is it differentially restricted? 1b) If restricted, is it restricted by specific individual or by role? 1c) Who defines roles in the institution, and who decides what access is appropriate for each role? 1d) How are appropriate access privileges determined? 1e) Are temporary employees given access to systems? If so, how? Who grants that access?

2a) Do users have access to all patient records? 2b) If so, how do you regulate cross-patient queries? 2c) Is access granted or denied to the entire medical record, or is the record segmented and access granted to segments? 2d) If segmented, who defines these segments and decides access policy to them? Is it the information systems department, a medical records committee, . . . ?

3a) Is restriction of access to medical records preemptive, or is presumptive access granted with audit based review? 3b) How do you monitor staff access to other resources? 3c) Is there a regular report generated on access requests and access grants/denials?

4a) Are certain types of records kept more secure (field limitations on HIV lab tests, VIP records, etc.)? 4b) Are psychiatric records on-line? If so are they treated specially for access? 4c) Is HIV status on-line. Is it treated specially for access? Is HIV infection or AIDS suppressed from the problem list? 4d) Are medication lists altered to hide HIV or psychiatric medications?

D. Encryption

1a) Are databases encrypted? If so, what type of encryption is used? If not, are databases protected only through access control?

2a) Are data encrypted during transmission over the network or to remote sites? If so, what type of encryption is used?

E. Protection Against External Threats

1a) What mechanisms are used to secure access from outside the institution? Dial-back schemes? Firewalls? Private lines or public networks? Authentication schemes? Encryption techniques?

2a) Are mechanisms in place to detect outsider probes? How do you know if someone is "sniffing" your system? 2b) Are there technical means available for detecting intrusion? 2c) What administrative mechanisms are used (awareness, reporting mechanisms, etc.)?

F. Software Discipline

1a) What types of software controls are in place to protect against Trojan horses and viruses?

2a) How do you attempt to control/limit the copying of data to prevent its subsequent release or unauthorized use?

G. Backup Procedures

1a) Do you have procedures in place for regularly backing up computer data? 1b) If so, what data are backed up: medical records, administrative data, password and access files? 1c) How frequently are data backed up and by whom? 1d) Where are backup tapes stored? 1e) Are back-up data stored in an encrypted or unencrypted form?

H. Emergencies/Contingency Plans

1a) What types of backup systems are in place to restore information/service in case of a catastrophe: redundancy, data storage, networks?

2a) How do you handle contingency/disaster planning? 2b) Are there formal procedures in place? 2c) Is there an oversight committee?

XI. User perspectives

A1) How important do users believe privacy and security are in health information systems? A2) What input did/do they have into the choice of security measures used or the design of the information system? A3) Do most users tend to favor or promote systems that require the least additional effort on their part? A4) Would users likely be strong supporters of increased security systems, or reluctant participants in systems that add to their daily workload? A5) What particular challenges did user perspectives add to the design process?

B1) Do users utilize the systems as intended? B2) Do they understand the security systems that are in place? B3) Do they find them effective? B4) Have they found ways to circumvent security measures that they don't believe provide real value? B5) What changes do users believe would make the system more effective and user friendly?

C1) Have security measures had adverse effects on the provision of health care? C2) Have there been cases in which physicians were unable to access an electronic record, or accessed wrong information, which caused a bad outcome? C3) How do security measures affect the availability of systems/information? C4) Have security measures resulted in denial of services?

D1) Do physicians and nurses put different types of information into an electronic patient record than they would put into a paper record? D2) If clinical notes are dictated, what confidentiality provisions apply to the transcription service? D3) Is it in-house or not? D4) Are there policies that cover dictation? D5) How are they enforced?

XII. Future research/needs

A1) How well have existing security measures worked? A2) What threats are not addressed or incompletely addressed? A3) What types of enhancements could be made to existing systems? A4) What would you do next if additional funding was made available for system upgrades?

B1) What types of incentives are necessary to stimulate adoption of additional security measures? B2) What is necessary to give other organizations the incentive to adopt electronic medical records and adequate security mechanisms?

C1) How will the perceived threat change over time? How will countermeasures change?

D1) How will future development of information technology change the privacy and security picture? D2) Does the prospect of computers in the home imply significant changes or challenges to your current operations?

E1) What technologies do you know of that are currently under development that could have a significant impact on system security and accessibility?

APPENDIX
B
Individuals Who Briefed the Study Committee

Joshua S. Auerbach, IBM T.J. Watson Research Center
Kit Bakke, Group Health Cooperative of Puget Sound
Glenda Barnes, Cylink Corporation
Paul Billings, Veterans Administration, Palo Alto Health Care Center
William R. Braithwaite, U.S. Department of Health and Human Services
Patricia L. Branum, Merck-Medco Inc.
A.G. Breitenstein, JRI Health Associates
Jean Chenowith, HCIA Inc.
James S. Corbett, Medical Information Bureau Inc.
Neil Day, Medical Information Bureau Inc.
Donald E. Detmer, University of Virginia
Gary Dickinson, Health Data Sciences Corporation
John P. Fanning, U.S. Department of Health and Human Services
Hansjürgen Garstka, Berlin Data Commission
Janlori Goldman, Center for Democracy and Technology
Donald Haines, American Civil Liberties Union
Isaac S. Kohane, Children's Hospital, Boston
Terry S. Latanich, Merck-Medco Inc.
John Lauer, Health Data Sciences Corporation
Donald A. Lindberg, National Library of Medicine
William H. Murray, Deloitte and Touche, LLP
Gary S. Persinger, Pharmaceutical Research and Manufacturers of
    America
Marc Rotenberg, Electronic Privacy Information Center
H. Jeffrey Smith, Georgetown University
Burt Tregub, Cylink Corporation
Daniel C. Walden, Merck-Medco Inc.

C

National Library of Medicine Awards to Develop Health Care Applications of the National Information Infrastructure

On October 7, 1996, Secretary of Health and Human Services Donna E. Shalala announced that the National Library of Medicine (NLM), a part of the National Institutes of Health, was funding 19 projects with a total budget of $42 million to develop health care applications of the national information infrastructure. The multiyear projects, located in 13 states and the District of Columbia, will serve as models for evaluating the impact of telemedicine[1] applications on cost, quality, and access to health care; assessing various approaches to ensuring the confidentiality of health data transmitted via electronic networks; and testing emerging health data standards. The Agency for Health Care Policy and Research is co-funding one of the 19 projects. The following project summaries are derived from a list of project descriptions prepared by NLM and are available on-line at nlm.nih.gov/research/initprojsum.html.

FUNDED PROJECTS

1. **Provide health care to underserved center-city elderly and off-shore islanders in California.** The University of Southern California's Medical faculty will treat multiple underserved communities ranging from North Hollywood's center-city elderly and minorities to the rela-

---

[1]Telemedicine is the use of computers, the Internet, and other communications technologies to provide medical care to patients at a distance.

tively isolated offshore island of Catalina via state-of-the-art telemedicine systems. Patients will be cared for in their own locale by means of PacBell network transmittal of USC Emergency medicine support instead of having to travel to distant specialists (e.g., by helicopter or boat from Catalina).

Contact: F.W. George III, M.D.
University of Southern California
Advanced Biotechnical Consortium
1537 Norfolk Street, DEI-5103
Los Angeles, CA 90033
(213) 342-3671

2. **Support rural primary care physicians consulting with remote specialists in West Virginia**. A consortium of nine institutions led by the Concurrent Engineering Research Center of the West Virginia University will demonstrate the viability of secure clinical telemedicine on public telecommunication networks and show that its adoption as an integral part of an overall health care plan can result in cost savings and improved access to quality health care for rural populations. Rural primary care physicians, physicians' assistants, and other authorized users will have secure access to electronic medical records and patient monitor data, and be able to confer with collaborating health care providers at a distance in the treatment of patients.

Contact: Ramana Reddy, Ph.D.
Concurrent Engineering Research Center
West Virginia University
886 Chestnut Ridge Road
Morgantown, WV 26506
(304) 293-7226 (304) 293-7541(fax)

3. **Improve care to high-risk newborns and their families in Massachusetts**. Beth Israel Deaconess Medical Center will use telemedicine to provide educational and emotional support to families of high-risk newborns both during their hospitalization and following discharge. This innovative use of technology should increase parents understanding of their baby's continuing medical needs and provide a clear cost savings. Prior to their baby's discharge from the hospital, parents will be able to observe the baby's care via a television monitor in their home. Following discharge, patients in their homes will continue to be connected via television to Beth Israel Hospital. The trial will examine the potential of

telemedicine to decrease the cost of care for very-low-birth-weight infants by increasing the efficiency of care.

Contact: Charles Safran, M.D.
Principal Investigator
Beth Israel Deaconess Medical Center
350 Longwood Avenue
Boston, MA 02115
(617) 732-5925

4. **Test real-time transmission of vital sign data from patients in ambulances to a hospital trauma center in Maryland.** BDM Federal Inc. and the University of Maryland at Baltimore will develop an advanced mobile telemedicine testbed that will investigate the feasibility and practicality of transmitting real-time vital sign data and video images of patients from inside the ambulance to the hospital's trauma center and clinical information system via cellular communications and local area network technology. The purpose of the mobile testbed is to improve the quality and timeliness of care provided during the "golden hour" and to provide better information to the emergency room (ER) staff prior to the arrival of patients in the ER. If proven feasible, this mobile telemedicine application could be used in trauma centers throughout the United States.

Contact: David Gagliano
BDM Federal Inc.
1501 BDM Way
McLean, VA 22102
(703) 848-6134

5. **Improve disease prevention and manage chronic illnesses in home settings in New York.** Columbia University will use technology to provide information to patients to improve disease prevention activities and effectively manage chronic illnesses in the home setting. Patients will receive alerts and reminders when standards of care (immunization, diabetes management, asthma control, etc.) are not being achieved. Patients will enter data (blood pressures, glucose levels, pulmonary function test results, etc.) into an electronic medical record using applications that run on home-based personal computers connected to the national information infrastructure (NII). These patients will also be able to communicate with health care providers, review their medical records, and receive desired information that will address their specific health care concerns. The project will demonstrate techniques to safeguard the confidentiality of personal health care records that are stored and transmitted electroni-

cally, and will evaluate the impact of patient use of information via the NII.

Contact: Soumitra Sengupta, Ph.D.
Assistant Professor
Department of Medical Informatics
Columbia University
161 Fort Washington Avenue
New York, NY 10032
(212) 305-7035

6. **Prevent adverse drug interactions among the elderly in Missouri**. Adverse drug interactions are often a problem, particularly among the elderly and others who take multiple medications. Sometimes the wrong dosage makes a medication more harmful than beneficial. But in St. Louis, and neighboring towns in Illinois, six hospitals are learning to prevent these problems, using the extensive telemedicine network that already links them. By year's end, they will be able to ensure that patients are taking the correct dosage of their medications, and to prevent or quickly respond to harmful drug events. Using pharmacy orders and patient data such as age, sex and weight, DoseChecker examines the prescriptions a patient is taking and issues dosage warnings when warranted. The other system, the Adverse Drug Event (ADE) Monitor, pulls together patient drug orders and laboratory test results, alerting hospital pharmacists when it detects signs of adverse reactions. Doctors and other health professionals will be notified immediately when a patient is at risk. This project was co-funded by the Agency for Health Care Policy and Research.

Contact: Michael Kahn, M.D.
Barnes-Jewish Hospital
216 South Kings Highway
St. Louis, MO 63110
(314) 454-8651

7. **Provide vital health information to health professionals in rural and urban settings across the Northwest**. The University of Washington Academic Medical Center regional telemedicine network will connect health professionals and patients from big cities, small towns, and vast expanses of sparsely populated areas in Washington, Wyoming, Alaska, Montana, and Idaho to provide timely access to vital health information. The University of Washington links clinical and public health partners at selected sites in this five-state area via a regional telemedicine network

that includes a World Wide Web interface to electronic medical records; secure clinical e-mail for clinician-to-clinician and clinician-to-patient interactions; electronic delivery and management of x-rays and other clinical images; and access to medical library resources, such as MEDLINE and full-text journals. This innovative network will allow clinicians to consult with one another, health professionals and their patients to confer, and all to access medical information, despite the long distances that separate them.

Contact: Sherrilynne Fuller, Ph.D.
University of Washington
A-327 Health Sciences Center
Box 356340
Seattle, WA 98195-6340
(206) 616-5808

8. **Provide patients with access to their own medical records while preserving confidentiality of that information in California.** In a cooperative effort with the Science Applications International Corporation (SAIC), the University of California, San Diego has launched PCASSO, a project designed to enable patients, health care providers, and medical researchers to access clinical information over the Internet without any breaches of confidentiality. PCASSO will use everyday World Wide Web technology to support information search and retrieval, and state-of-the-art security technology to ensure patient privacy and the integrity of patient information. The project represents a new thrust within the health care industry: to provide patients more control over and access to their own medical records while preserving the confidentiality of that information.

Contact: Dixie Baker, M.D.
Science Applications International Corporation
10260 Campus Point Drive
San Diego, CA 92121
(310) 615-0305

9. **Transmit and manage brain and breast images and associated medical data in four California medical centers**. This project, coordinated by the Department of Radiology at the University of California at San Francisco, is focused in scope but may prove to have far-reaching consequences for health care delivery. It links four San Francisco-area medical centers electronically, for the transmission and management of neuroradiology and mammography images. The hope is that a high-

performance tele-imaging information infrastructure will enhance health care in the Bay Area by improving telediagnosis, teleconsultation, tele-management, teleresearch, and tele-education. Then, perhaps, this model can be extended to include other types of medical images, and other parts of the country.

Contact: H.K. Huang, D.Sc.
University of California, San Francisco
Department of Radiology
School of Medicine
530 Parnassus Avenue, RM CL-158
San Francisco, CA 94143-0628
(415) 476-6044

10. **Measure the effectiveness of video consultations for patients with special needs, including children with disabilities or heart conditions and persons with mental illness in Iowa.** The University of Iowa's National Laboratory for the Study of Rural Telemedicine was created in 1994. Now, with support from NLM, that group will expand its efforts in two directions: clinical consultations and the use of specialized databases in health care delivery. A series of projects will measure the effectiveness of video consultations for patients with special needs, including children with disabilities or heart conditions and persons with mental illness. Another project will give community hospital emergency rooms access to information and expertise by providing special database software and allowing teleconferencing with physicians at the University of Iowa Health Center. NLM funding will also support an innovative project to deliver health information into the homes of people with diabetes. They will receive an easy-to-use device that attaches to their TV and provides access to on-line health information. Researchers hope that this project will help diabetes patients manage their disease more effectively.

Contact: Michael Kienzle, M.D.
University of Iowa
National Laboratory for the Study of Rural Telemedicine
Telemedicine Resource Center
1-204 MEB
Iowa City, IA 52242
(319) 353-5621

11. **Analyze the benefits of rural telemedicine services by linking health professionals in three small Missouri communities.** The University of Missouri-Columbia School of Medicine will implement and then

analyze the benefits of rural telemedicine services, working with three small rural Missouri communities. In addition to creating links among the health professionals in each community, the project will connect rural providers to colleagues in other participating towns and to the university's Health Sciences Center, with its four hospitals, extensive medical library, hundreds of specialists, and other resources. Studies will involve tracking utilization of this new network, assessing rural providers' needs, and noting any changes in health care utilization patterns and retention of health care personnel in rural communities after the network is in place. Costs of and savings from this venture will also be carefully reviewed.

Contact: Joyce A. Mitchell, Ph.D.
University of Missouri-Columbia
School of Medicine
Medical Informatics Group
605 Lewis Hall
Columbia, MO 65211
(573) 884-7717

12. **Expand robust health care network that provides rapid access to patient record data in Indiana.** With new funding from the NLM, Indiana University School of Medicine will broaden the scope of its existing Indianapolis Network for Health Care of hospital emergency rooms, clinics, HMOs, homeless care sites, and pharmacies, so that more people can enjoy its benefits. Already this technically robust network provides instant access to patient records in emergency rooms and efficient access to medical library resources at numerous care sites, and permits collection of prescription information from a large chain of community pharmacies, to improve drug prescribing patterns in a range of health care facilities. New network linkages will include the Indiana State Public Health Department and a number of large clinical laboratories. Among other benefits, these additions to the network will provide clinicians on the network with better immunization data from health departments and will enable electronic reporting of communicable diseases from high-volume Marion County clinical laboratories to the relevant public health departments.

Contact: Clement J. McDonald, M.D.
Indiana University, Regenstrief Institute
Department of Medicine
1001 W 10th Street, Fifth Floor
Indianapolis, IN 46202-2859
(317) 630-7400

13. **Provide health care teams with computer systems to assist in outpatient care in Illinois.** The goal of Northwestern Memorial Hospital's NetReach project is to provide health care teams with computer systems to assist in outpatient care, and to evaluate the impact of their use. The project observed practicing clinicians at seven diverse outpatient clinics (primary care, specialty care, faculty group practice, independent group practice, and urban care clinics) to understand and specify the information needs of clinicians. Based on the requirements derived from the information needs study, they implemented information tools, including a computer-based patient record at one site, to address the clinicians' needs. During the NLM-funded extension, the project will evaluate the impact of information technology on clinical and operational performance of physicians and on patient and provider satisfaction.

Contact: Paul Tang, M.D.
Northwestern Memorial Hospital
Information Services
259 East Erie, Suite 600
Chicago, IL 60611
(312) 908-4034

14. **Increase the efficiency and improve the quality of emergency room and primary care in Indiana.** The Indiana University School of Medicine will create the Indianapolis Network for Patient Care, a shared clinical data repository that will store encounter records, hospital abstracts, clinical laboratory data, prescription data, and other data for use by emergency room departments and primary care providers in the Indianapolis area. This repository will encompass 90 percent of Indianapolis's hospital emergency room care data and data from two managed-care systems, as well as a major share of the laboratory and hospital encounter data of the city. The purpose of this effort will be to increase the efficiency and improve the quality of emergency room care and primary care by providing the responsible physicians with laboratory and other data important to care. The completion of this project should result in a workable model for access and confidentiality for large-scale shared community clinical data.

Contact: Clement J. McDonald, M.D.
Indiana University, Regenstrief Institute
Department of Medicine
1001 W 10th Street, Fifth Floor
Indianapolis, IN 46202-2859
(317) 630-7400

15. **Provide telemedicine services to renal dialysis patients and information services for caregivers in the District of Columbia.** Georgetown University Medical Center already has an extensive network consisting of radiological imaging nodes and hospital information systems that provide support to the nephrologists at the medical center and at home. The network links Georgetown University Medical Center, remote outpatient kidney dialysis clinics, and nephrologists' homes. The primary functions of the network are to provide telemedicine services to renal dialysis patients, to create, manage, transfer, and use electronic health data and to provide decision support and information services for caregivers. This project will test the general hypothesis that by facilitating electronic interactive communication among physicians and patients, quality of patient care will be improved and lower costs to patients, physicians, and the health care system will be incurred.

Contact: Seong Ki Mun, Ph.D.
Georgetown University Medical Center
37th and O Streets, N.W.
Washington, DC 20057
(202) 784-3483

16. **Establish a network for prevention and health care in Massachusetts.** Increased access to information resources and technology allows consumers to take greater responsibility for health and wellness, as well as for their own health care. Boston College and the Partners HealthCare System will examine the impact of public education and access to information on matters of lifestyle and health; patient access to information about specific health problems; support for health care providers for facilitating optimal care practices; and clinical services provided by the health care system.

Contact: Robert A. Greenes, M.D.
Brigham and Women's Hospital
75 Francis Street
Boston, MA 02115
(617) 732-6281

17. **Evaluate the impact of telemedicine technologies and applications on the health care system in rural Alaska.** As federal health care contributions to health care systems decrease, and as the population of Alaska changes, telemedicine is seen as a strategy for cost containment and for increasing the quality of health care delivery that, in Alaska, has traditionally relied on the transportation of patients over long distances.

The objective of this project is to replicate existing and developed Alaska telemedicine testbeds by modifying, interfacing, and expanding successfully deployed telemedicine technologies and to evaluate the impact of these technologies on the health care system in rural Alaska for cost, quality of care, and access to care by rural Native Alaskans where and when it is needed.

Contact: Frederick W. Pearce, Ph.D.
University of Alaska Anchorage
Applied Science Laboratory
3211 Providence Drive
Anchorage, AK 99508
(907) 786-4183

18. **Use teledermatology to improve the ability of primary care physicians to recognize and treat skin cancers and other skin conditions in Oregon.** This extension of an NLM contract at the Oregon Health Sciences University in Portland, Oregon, will expand the range of technologies used to provide remote dermatologic diagnosis and will collect and analyze data on teledermatology's impact on the quality and cost of health care.

Contact: Douglas A. Perednia, M.D.
Oregon Health Sciences University
3181 SW Sam Jackson Park Road
Portland, OR 97201
(503) 494-6846

19. **Improve the quality and efficiency of patient care by providing physicians with rapid access to important clinical information in a single, easy-to-use workstation environment in Pennsylvania.** An extension of an NLM contact at the University of Pittsburgh will evaluate the clinical utility of a multimedia clinical information system at the University of Pittsburgh's Cancer Institute. Currently, the system can acquire, compress, store, retrieve, display, and manipulate many kinds of clinical images, including radiographs, CT scans, nuclear medicine studies, gastrointestinal endoscopy images, EKGs, and microscopic pathology. These images are linked, in real-time, with a wide range of clinical reports stored in the University of Pittsburgh Medical Center's electronic medical record system. The project will study the effect of integrated access to clinical images and textual patient data on the length of time required to diagnose cancer and on the management of cancer treatment.

Contact: Henry J. Lowe, M.D.
Section on Medical Informatics
University of Pittsburgh
B50A Lothrop Hall
Pittsburgh, PA 15261
(412) 648-3190

D

Sections of the Health Insurance Portability and Accountability Act of 1996 (Public Law 104-191) Related to the Privacy and Security of Electronic Health Information

TITLE II—PREVENTING HEALTH CARE FRAUD AND ABUSE; ADMINISTRATIVE SIMPLIFICATION

Subtitle F—Administrative Simplification

SEC. 261. PURPOSE.

It is the purpose of this subtitle to improve the Medicare program under title XVIII of the Social Security Act, the medicaid program under title XIX of such Act, and the efficiency and effectiveness of the health care system, by encouraging the development of a health information system through the establishment of standards and requirements for the electronic transmission of certain health information.

SEC. 262. ADMINISTRATIVE SIMPLIFICATION.

(a) IN GENERAL.—Title XI (42 U.S.C. 1301 et seq.) is amended by adding at the end the following:

"PART C—ADMINISTRATIVE SIMPLIFICATION
"DEFINITIONS
"SEC. 1171. For purposes of this part:

NOTE: The material reproduced in this appendix has been reprinted from an electronic version of the Congressional Record—House, July 31, 1996, H9495-H9499. It is intended for use as a general reference, and not for legal research or other work requiring authenticated primary sources.

"(1) CODE SET.—The term 'code set' means any set of codes used for encoding data elements, such as tables of terms, medical concepts, medical diagnostic codes, or medical procedure codes.

"(2) HEALTH CARE CLEARINGHOUSE.—The term 'health care clearinghouse' means a public or private entity that processes or facilitates the processing of nonstandard data elements of health information into standard data elements.

"(3) HEALTH CARE PROVIDER.—The term 'health care provider' includes a provider of services (as defined in section 1861(u)), a provider of medical or other health services (as defined in section 1861(s)), and any other person furnishing health care services or supplies.

"(4) HEALTH INFORMATION.—The term 'health information' means any information, whether oral or recorded in any form or medium, that—

"(A) is created or received by a health care provider, health plan, public health authority, employer, life insurer, school or university, or health care clearinghouse; and

"(B) relates to the past, present, or future physical or mental health or condition of an individual, the provision of health care to an individual, or the past, present, or future payment for the provision of health care to an individual.

"(5) HEALTH PLAN.—The term 'health plan' means an individual or group plan that provides, or pays the cost of, medical care (as such term is defined in section 2791 of the Public Health Service Act). Such term includes the following, and any combination thereof:

"(A) A group health plan (as defined in section 2791(a) of the Public Health Service Act), but only if the plan—

"(i) has 50 or more participants (as defined in section 3(7) of the Employee Retirement Income Security Act of 1974); or

"(ii) is administered by an entity other than the employer who established and maintains the plan.

"(B) A health insurance issuer (as defined in section 2791(b) of the Public Health Service Act).

"(C) A health maintenance organization (as defined in section 2791(b) of the Public Health Service Act).

"(D) Part A or part B of the Medicare program under title XVIII.

"(E) The medicaid program under title XIX.

"(F) A Medicare supplemental policy (as defined in section 1882(g)(1)).

"(G) A long-term care policy, including a nursing home fixed indemnity policy (unless the Secretary determines that such a policy does not provide sufficiently comprehensive coverage of a benefit so that the policy should be treated as a health plan).

"(H) An employee welfare benefit plan or any other arrangement which is established or maintained for the purpose of offering or providing health benefits to the employees of 2 or more employers.

"(I) The health care program for active military personnel under title 10, United States Code.

"(J) The veterans health care program under chapter 17 of title 38, United States Code.

"(K) The Civilian Health and Medical Program of the Uniformed Services (CHAMPUS), as defined in section 1072(4) of title 10, United States Code.

"(L) The Indian health service program under the Indian Health Care Improvement Act (25 U.S.C. 1601 et seq.).

"(M) The Federal Employees Health Benefit Plan under chapter 89 of title 5, United States Code.

"(6) INDIVIDUALLY IDENTIFIABLE HEALTH INFORMATION.—The term 'individually identifiable health information' means any information, including demographic information collected from an individual, that—

"(A) is created or received by a health care provider, health plan, employer, or health care clearinghouse; and

"(B) relates to the past, present, or future physical or mental health or condition of an individual, the provision of health care to an individual, or the past, present, or future payment for the provision of health care to an individual, and—

"(i) identifies the individual; or

"(ii) with respect to which there is a reasonable basis to believe that the information can be used to identify the individual.

"(7) STANDARD.—The term 'standard', when used with reference to a data element of health information or a transaction referred to in section 1173(a)(1), means any such data element or transaction that meets each of the standards and implementation specifications adopted or established by the Secretary with respect to the data element or transaction under sections 1172 through 1174.

"(8) STANDARD SETTING ORGANIZATION.—The term 'standard setting organization' means a standard setting organization accredited by the American National Standards Institute, including the National Council for Prescription Drug Programs, that develops standards for information transactions, data elements, or any other standard that is necessary to, or will facilitate, the implementation of this part.

"GENERAL REQUIREMENTS FOR ADOPTION OF STANDARDS

"SEC. 1172. (a) APPLICABILITY.—Any standard adopted under this part shall apply, in whole or in part, to the following persons:

"(1) A health plan.

"(2) A health care clearinghouse.

"(3) A health care provider who transmits any health information in electronic form in connection with a transaction referred to in section 1173(a)(1).

"(b) REDUCTION OF COSTS.—Any standard adopted under this part shall be consistent with the objective of reducing the administrative costs of providing and paying for health care.

"(c) ROLE OF STANDARD SETTING ORGANIZATIONS.—

"(1) IN GENERAL.—Except as provided in paragraph (2), any standard adopted under this part shall be a standard that has been developed, adopted, or modified by a standard setting organization.

"(2) SPECIAL RULES.—

"(A) DIFFERENT STANDARDS.—The Secretary may adopt a standard that is different from any standard developed, adopted, or modified by a standard setting organization, if—

"(i) the different standard will substantially reduce administrative costs to health care providers and health plans compared to the alternatives; and

"(ii) the standard is promulgated in accordance with the rulemaking procedures of subchapter III of chapter 5 of title 5, United States Code.

"(B) NO STANDARD BY STANDARD SETTING ORGANIZATION.—If no standard setting organization has developed, adopted, or modified any standard relating to a standard that the Secretary is authorized or required to adopt under this part—

"(i) paragraph (1) shall not apply; and

"(ii) subsection (f) shall apply.

"(3) CONSULTATION REQUIREMENT.—

"(A) IN GENERAL.—A standard may not be adopted under this part unless—

"(i) in the case of a standard that has been developed, adopted, or modified by a standard organization, the organization consulted with each of the organizations described in subparagraph (B) in the course of such development, adoption, or modification; and

"(ii) in the case of any other standard, the Secretary, in complying with the requirements of subsection (f), consulted with each of the organizations described in subparagraph (B) before adopting the standard.

"(B) ORGANIZATIONS DESCRIBED.—The organizations referred to in subparagraph (A) are the following:

"(i) The National Uniform Billing Committee.

"(ii) The National Uniform Claim Committee.

"(iii) The Workgroup for Electronic Data Interchange.

"(iv) The American Dental Association.

"(d) IMPLEMENTATION SPECIFICATIONS.—The Secretary shall establish specifications for implementing each of the standards adopted under this part.

"(e) PROTECTION OF TRADE SECRETS.—Except as otherwise required by law, a standard adopted under this part shall not require disclosure of trade secrets or confidential commercial information by a person required to comply with this part.

"(f) ASSISTANCE TO THE SECRETARY.—In complying with the requirements of this part, the Secretary shall rely on the recommendations of the National Committee on Vital and Health Statistics established under section 306(k) of the Public Health Service Act (42 U.S.C. 242k(k)), and shall consult with appropriate Federal and State agencies and private organizations. The Secretary shall publish in the Federal Register any recommendation of the National Committee on Vital and Health Statistics regarding the adoption of a standard under this part.

"(g) APPLICATION TO MODIFICATIONS OF STANDARDS.—This section shall apply to a modification to a standard (including an addition to a standard) adopted under section 1174(b) in the same manner as it applies to an initial standard adopted under section 1174(a).

"STANDARDS FOR INFORMATION TRANSACTIONS AND DATA ELEMENTS

"SEC. 1173. (a) STANDARDS TO ENABLE ELECTRONIC EXCHANGE.—

"(1) IN GENERAL.—The Secretary shall adopt standards for transactions, and data elements for such transactions, to enable health information to be exchanged electronically, that are appropriate for—

"(A) the financial and administrative transactions described in paragraph (2); and

"(B) other financial and administrative transactions determined appropriate by the Secretary, consistent with the goals of improving the operation of the health care system and reducing administrative costs.

"(2) TRANSACTIONS.—The transactions referred to in paragraph (1)(A) are transactions with respect to the following:

"(A) Health claims or equivalent encounter information.

"(B) Health claims attachments.

"(C) Enrollment and disenrollment in a health plan.

"(D) Eligibility for a health plan.

"(E) Health care payment and remittance advice.

"(F) Health plan premium payments.

"(G) First report of injury.

"(H) Health claim status.

"(I) Referral certification and authorization.

"(3) ACCOMMODATION OF SPECIFIC PROVIDERS.—The standards adopted by the Secretary under paragraph (1) shall accommodate the needs of different types of health care providers.

"(b) UNIQUE HEALTH IDENTIFIERS.—

"(1) IN GENERAL.—The Secretary shall adopt standards providing for a standard unique health identifier for each individual, employer, health plan, and health care provider for use in the health care system. In carrying out the preceding sentence for each health plan and health care provider, the Secretary shall take into account multiple uses for identifiers and multiple locations and specialty classifications for health care providers.

"(2) USE OF IDENTIFIERS.—The standards adopted under paragraph (1) shall specify the purposes for which a unique health identifier may be used.

"(c) CODE SETS.—

"(1) IN GENERAL.—The Secretary shall adopt standards that—

"(A) select code sets for appropriate data elements for the transactions referred to in subsection (a)(1) from among the code sets that have been developed by private and public entities; or

"(B) establish code sets for such data elements if no code sets for the data elements have been developed.

"(2) DISTRIBUTION.—The Secretary shall establish efficient and low-cost procedures for distribution (including electronic distribution) of code sets and modifications made to such code sets under section 1174(b).

"(d) SECURITY STANDARDS FOR HEALTH INFORMATION.—

"(1) SECURITY STANDARDS.—The Secretary shall adopt security standards that—

"(A) take into account—

"(i) the technical capabilities of record systems used to maintain health information;

"(ii) the costs of security measures;

"(iii) the need for training persons who have access to health information;

"(iv) the value of audit trails in computerized record systems; and

"(v) the needs and capabilities of small health care providers and rural health care providers (as such providers are defined by the Secretary); and

"(B) ensure that a health care clearinghouse, if it is part of a larger organization, has policies and security procedures which isolate the activities of the health care clearinghouse with respect to processing information in a manner that prevents unauthorized access to such information by such larger organization.

"(2) SAFEGUARDS.—Each person described in section 1172(a) who maintains or transmits health information shall maintain reasonable and appropriate administrative, technical, and physical safeguards—

"(A) to ensure the integrity and confidentiality of the information;

"(B) to protect against any reasonably anticipated—

"(i) threats or hazards to the security or integrity of the information; and

"(ii) unauthorized uses or disclosures of the information; and

"(C) otherwise to ensure compliance with this part by the officers and employees of such person.

"(e) ELECTRONIC SIGNATURE.—

"(1) STANDARDS.—The Secretary, in coordination with the Secretary of Commerce, shall adopt standards specifying procedures for the electronic transmission and authentication of signatures with respect to the transactions referred to in subsection (a)(1).

"(2) EFFECT OF COMPLIANCE.—Compliance with the standards adopted under paragraph (1) shall be deemed to satisfy Federal and State statutory requirements for written signatures with respect to the transactions referred to in subsection (a)(1).

"(f) TRANSFER OF INFORMATION AMONG HEALTH PLANS.—The Secretary shall adopt standards for transferring among health plans appropriate standard data elements needed for the coordination of benefits, the sequential processing of claims, and other data elements for individuals who have more than one health plan.

"TIMETABLES FOR ADOPTION OF STANDARDS

"SEC. 1174. (a) INITIAL STANDARDS.—The Secretary shall carry out section 1173 not later than 18 months after the date of the enactment of the Health Insurance Portability and Accountability Act of 1996, except that standards relating to claims attachments shall be adopted not later than 30 months after such date.

"(b) ADDITIONS AND MODIFICATIONS TO STANDARDS.—

"(1) IN GENERAL.—Except as provided in paragraph (2), the Secretary shall review the standards adopted under section 1173, and shall adopt modifications to the standards (including additions to the standards), as determined appropriate, but not more frequently than once every 12 months. Any addition or modification to a standard shall be completed in a manner which minimizes the disruption and cost of compliance.

"(2) SPECIAL RULES.—

"(A) FIRST 12-MONTH PERIOD.—Except with respect to additions and modifications to code sets under subparagraph (B), the Secretary may not adopt any modification to a standard adopted under this part during the 12-month period beginning on the date the standard is initially adopted, unless the Secretary determines that the modification is necessary in order to permit compliance with the standard.

"(B) ADDITIONS AND MODIFICATIONS TO CODE SETS.—

"(i) IN GENERAL.—The Secretary shall ensure that procedures exist for the routine maintenance, testing, enhancement, and expansion of code sets.

"(ii) ADDITIONAL RULES.—If a code set is modified under this subsection, the modified code set shall include instructions on how data elements of health information that were encoded prior to the modification may be converted or translated so as to preserve the informational value of the data elements that existed before the modification. Any modification to a code set under this subsection shall be implemented in a manner that minimizes the disruption and cost of complying with such modification.

"REQUIREMENTS

"SEC. 1175. (a) CONDUCT OF TRANSACTIONS BY PLANS.—

"(1) IN GENERAL.—If a person desires to conduct a transaction referred to in section 1173(a)(1) with a health plan as a standard transaction—

"(A) the health plan may not refuse to conduct such transaction as a standard transaction;

"(B) the insurance plan may not delay such transaction, or otherwise adversely affect, or attempt to adversely affect, the person or the transaction on the ground that the transaction is a standard transaction; and

"(C) the information transmitted and received in connection with the transaction shall be in the form of standard data elements of health information.

"(2) SATISFACTION OF REQUIREMENTS.—A health plan may satisfy the requirements under paragraph (1) by—

"(A) directly transmitting and receiving standard data elements of health information; or

"(B) submitting nonstandard data elements to a health care clearinghouse for processing into standard data elements and transmission by the health care clearinghouse, and receiving standard data elements through the health care clearinghouse.

"(3) TIMETABLE FOR COMPLIANCE.—Paragraph (1) shall not be construed to require a health plan to comply with any standard, implementation specification, or modification to a standard or specification adopted or established by the Secretary under sections 1172 through 1174 at any time prior to the date on which the plan is required to comply with the standard or specification under subsection (b).

"(b) COMPLIANCE WITH STANDARDS.—

"(1) INITIAL COMPLIANCE.—

"(A) IN GENERAL.—Not later than 24 months after the date on which an initial standard or implementation specification is adopted or established under sections 1172 and 1173, each person to whom the standard or implementation specification applies shall comply with the standard or specification.

"(B) SPECIAL RULE FOR SMALL HEALTH PLANS.—In the case of a small health plan, paragraph (1) shall be applied by substituting '36 months' for '24 months'. For purposes of this subsection, the Secretary shall determine the plans that qualify as small health plans.

"(2) COMPLIANCE WITH MODIFIED STANDARDS.—If the Secretary adopts a modification to a standard or implementation specification under this part, each person to whom the standard or implementation specification applies shall comply with the modified standard or implementation specification at such time as the Secretary determines appropriate, taking into account the time needed to comply due to the nature and extent of the modification. The time determined appropriate under the preceding sentence may not be earlier than the last day of the 180-day period beginning on the date such modification is adopted. The Secretary may extend the time for compliance for small health plans, if the Secretary determines that such extension is appropriate.

"(3) CONSTRUCTION.—Nothing in this subsection shall be construed to prohibit any person from complying with a standard or specification by—

"(A) submitting nonstandard data elements to a health care clearinghouse for processing into standard data elements and transmission by the health care clearinghouse; or

"(B) receiving standard data elements through a health care clearinghouse.

"GENERAL PENALTY FOR FAILURE TO COMPLY WITH
REQUIREMENTS AND STANDARDS

"SEC. 1176. (a) GENERAL PENALTY.—

"(1) IN GENERAL.—Except as provided in subsection (b), the Secretary shall impose on any person who violates a provision of this part a penalty of not more than $100 for each such violation, except that the total amount imposed on the person for all violations of an identical requirement or prohibition during a calendar year may not exceed $25,000.

"(2) PROCEDURES.—The provisions of section 1128A (other than subsections (a) and (b) and the second sentence of subsection (f)) shall apply to the imposition of a civil money penalty under this subsection in the same manner as such provisions apply to the imposition of a penalty under such section 1128A.

"(b) LIMITATIONS.—

"(1) OFFENSES OTHERWISE PUNISHABLE.—A penalty may not be imposed under subsection (a) with respect to an act if the act constitutes an offense punishable under section 1177.

"(2) NONCOMPLIANCE NOT DISCOVERED.—A penalty may not be imposed under subsection (a) with respect to a provision of this part if it is established to the satisfaction of the Secretary that the person liable for the penalty did not know, and by exercising reasonable diligence would not have known, that such person violated the provision.

"(3) FAILURES DUE TO REASONABLE CAUSE.—

"(A) IN GENERAL.—Except as provided in subparagraph (B), a penalty may not be imposed under subsection (a) if—

"(i) the failure to comply was due to reasonable cause and not to willful neglect; and

"(ii) the failure to comply is corrected during the 30-day period beginning on the first date the person liable for the penalty knew, or by exercising reasonable diligence would have known, that the failure to comply occurred.

"(B) EXTENSION OF PERIOD.—

"(i) NO PENALTY.—The period referred to in subparagraph (A)(ii) may be extended as determined appropriate by the Secretary based on the nature and extent of the failure to comply.

"(ii) ASSISTANCE.—If the Secretary determines that a person failed to comply because the person was unable to comply, the Secretary may provide technical assistance to the person during the period described in subparagraph (A)(ii). Such assistance shall be provided in any manner determined appropriate by the Secretary.

"(4) REDUCTION.—In the case of a failure to comply which is due to reasonable cause and not to willful neglect, any penalty under subsection (a) that is not entirely waived under paragraph (3) may be waived to the extent that the payment of such penalty would be excessive relative to the compliance failure involved.

"WRONGFUL DISCLOSURE OF INDIVIDUALLY IDENTIFIABLE HEALTH INFORMATION

"SEC. 1177. (a) OFFENSE.—A person who knowingly and in violation of this part—

"(1) uses or causes to be used a unique health identifier;

"(2) obtains individually identifiable health information relating to an individual; or

"(3) discloses individually identifiable health information to another person, shall be punished as provided in subsection (b).

"(b) PENALTIES.—A person described in subsection (a) shall—

"(1) be fined not more than $50,000, imprisoned not more than 1 year, or both;

"(2) if the offense is committed under false pretenses, be fined not more than $100,000, imprisoned not more than 5 years, or both; and

"(3) if the offense is committed with intent to sell, transfer, or use individually identifiable health information for commercial advantage, personal gain, or malicious harm, be fined not more than $250,000, imprisoned not more than 10 years, or both.

"EFFECTS ON STATE LAW

"SEC. 1178. (a) GENERAL EFFECT.—

"(1) GENERAL RULE.—Except as provided in paragraph (2), a provision or requirement under this part, or a standard or implementation specification adopted or established under sections 1172 through 1174, shall supersede any contrary provision of State law, including a provision of State law that requires medical or health plan records (including billing information) to bemaintained or transmitted in written rather than electronic form.

"(2) EXCEPTIONS.—A provision or requirement under this part, or a standard or implementation specification adopted or established under sections 1172 through 1174, shall not supersede a contrary provision of State law, if the provision of State law—

"(A) is a provision the Secretary determines—

"(i) is necessary—

"(I) to prevent fraud and abuse;

"(II) to ensure appropriate State regulation of insurance and health plans;

"(III) for State reporting on health care delivery or costs; or

"(IV) for other purposes; or

"(ii) addresses controlled substances; or

"(B) subject to section 264(c)(2) of the Health Insurance Portability and Accountability Act of 1996, relates to the privacy of individually identifiable health information.

"b) PUBLIC HEALTH.—Nothing in this part shall be construed to invalidate or limit the authority, power, or procedures established under any law providing for the reporting of disease or injury, child abuse, birth, or death, public health surveillance, or public health investigation or intervention.

"(c) STATE REGULATORY REPORTING.—Nothing in this part shall limit the ability of a State to require a health plan to report, or to provide access to, information for management audits, financial audits, program monitoring and evaluation, facility licensure or certification, or individual licensure or certification.

"PROCESSING PAYMENT TRANSACTIONS BY FINANCIAL INSTITUTIONS

"SEC. 1179. To the extent that an entity is engaged in activities of a financial institution (as defined in section 1101 of the Right to Financial Privacy Act of 1978), or is engaged in authorizing, processing, clearing, settling, billing, transferring, reconciling, or collecting payments, for a financial institution, this part, and any standard adopted under this part, shall not apply to the entity with respect to such activities, including the following:

"(1) The use or disclosure of information by the entity for authorizing, processing, clearing, settling, billing, transferring, reconciling or collecting, a payment for, or related to, health plan premiums or health care, where such payment is made by any means, including a credit, debit, or other payment card, an account, check, or electronic funds transfer.

"(2) The request for, or the use or disclosure of, information by the entity with respect to a payment described in paragraph (1)—

"(A) for transferring receivables;

"(B) for auditing;

"(C) in connection with—

"(i) a customer dispute; or

"(ii) an inquiry from, or to, a customer;

"(D) in a communication to a customer of the entity regarding the customer's transactions, payment card, account, check, or electronic funds transfer;

"(E) for reporting to consumer reporting agencies; or

"(F) for complying with—

"(i) a civil or criminal subpoena; or

"(ii) a Federal or State law regulating the entity.".

(b) CONFORMING AMENDMENTS.—

(1) REQUIREMENT FOR MEDICARE PROVIDERS.—Section 1866(a)(1)(42 U.S.C.

1395cc(a)(1)) is amended—

(A) by striking 'and' at the end of subparagraph (P);

(B) by striking the period at the end of subparagraph (Q) and inserting "; and"; and

(C) by inserting immediately after subparagraph (Q) the following new subparagraph:

"(R) to contract only with a health care clearinghouse (as defined in section 1171) that meets each standard and implementation specification adopted or established under part C of title XI on or after the date on which the health care clearinghouse is required to comply with the standard or specification.".

(2) TITLE HEADING.—Title XI (42 U.S.C. 1301 et seq.) is amended by striking the title heading and inserting the following:

"TITLE XI—GENERAL PROVISIONS, PEER REVIEW, AND ADMINISTRATIVE SIMPLIFICATION".

SEC. 263. CHANGES IN MEMBERSHIP AND DUTIES OF NATIONAL COMMITTEE ON VITAL AND HEALTH STATISTICS.

Section 306(k) of the Public Health Service Act (42 U.S.C. 242k(k)) is amended—

(1) in paragraph (1), by striking "16" and inserting "18";

(2) by amending paragraph (2) to read as follows:

"(2) The members of the Committee shall be appointed from among persons who have distinguished themselves in the fields of health statistics, electronic interchange of health care information, privacy and security of electronic information, population-based public health, purchasing or financing health care services, integrated computerized health information systems, health services research, consumer interests in health information, health data standards, epidemiology, and the provision of health services. Members of the Committee shall be appointed for terms of 4 years.";

(3) by redesignating paragraphs (3) through (5) as paragraphs (4) through (6), respectively, and inserting after paragraph (2) the following:

"(3) Of the members of the Committee—

"(A) 1 shall be appointed, not later than 60 days after the date of the enactment of the Health Insurance Portability and Accountability Act of 1996, by the Speaker of the House of Representatives after consultation with the Minority Leader of the House of Representatives;

"(B) 1 shall be appointed, not later than 60 days after the date of the enactment of the Health Insurance Portability and Accountability Act of 1996, by the

President pro tempore of the Senate after consultation with the Minority Leader of the Senate; and

"(C) 16 shall be appointed by the Secretary.";

(4) by amending paragraph (5) (as so redesignated) to read as follows:

"(5) The Committee—

"(A) shall assist and advise the Secretary—

"(i) to delineate statistical problems bearing on health and health services which are of national or international interest;

"(ii) to stimulate studies of such problems by other organizations and agencies whenever possible or to make investigations of such problems through subcommittees;

"(iii) to determine, approve, and revise the terms, definitions, classifications, and guidelines for assessing health status and health services, their distribution and costs, for use (I) within the Department of Health and Human Services, (II) by all programs administered or funded by the Secretary, including the Federal-State-local cooperative health statistics system referred to in subsection (e), and (III) to the extent possible as determined by the head of the agency involved, by the Department of Veterans Affairs, the Department of Defense, and other Federal agencies concerned with health and health services;

"(iv) with respect to the design of and approval of health statistical and health information systems concerned with the collection, processing, and tabulation of health statistics within the Department of Health and Human Services, with respect to the Cooperative Health Statistics System established under subsection (e), and with respect to the standardized means for the collection of health information and statistics to be established by the Secretary under subsection (j)(1);

"(v) to review and comment on findings and proposals developed by other organizations and agencies and to make recommendations for their adoption or implementation by local, State, national, or international agencies;

"(vi) to cooperate with national committees of other countries and with the World Health Organization and other national agencies in the studies of problems of mutual interest;

"(vii) to issue an annual report on the state of the Nation's health, its health services, their costs and distributions, and to make proposals for improvement of the Nation's health statistics and health information systems; and

"(viii) in complying with the requirements imposed on the Secretary under part C of title XI of the Social Security Act;

"(B) shall study the issues related to the adoption of uniform data standards for patient medical record information and the electronic exchange of such information;

"(C) shall report to the Secretary not later than 4 years after the date of the enactment of the Health Insurance Portability and Accountability Act of 1996 recommendations and legislative proposals for such standards and electronic exchange; and

"(D) shall be responsible generally for advising the Secretary and the Congress on the status of the implementation of part C of title XI of the Social Security Act."; and

(5) by adding at the end the following:

"(7) Not later than 1 year after the date of the enactment of the Health Insurance Portability and Accountability Act of 1996, and annually thereafter, the Committee shall submit to the Congress, and make public, a report regarding the implementation of part C of title XI of the Social Security Act. Such report shall address the following subjects, to the extent that the Committee determines appropriate:

"(A) The extent to which persons required to comply with part C of title XI of the Social Security Act are cooperating in implementing the standards adopted under such part.

"(B) The extent to which such entities are meeting the security standards adopted under such part and the types of penalties assessed for noncompliance with such standards.

"(C) Whether the Federal and State Governments are receiving information of sufficient quality to meet their responsibilities under such part.

"(D) Any problems that exist with respect to implementation of such part.

"(E) The extent to which timetables under such part are being met.".

SEC. 264. RECOMMENDATIONS WITH RESPECT TO PRIVACY OF CERTAIN HEALTH INFORMATION.

(a) IN GENERAL.—Not later than the date that is 12 months after the date of the enactment of this Act, the Secretary of Health and Human Services shall submit to the Committee on Labor and Human Resources and the Committee on Finance of the Senate and the Committee on Commerce and the Committee on Ways and Means of the House of Representatives detailed recommendations on standards with respect to the privacy of individually identifiable health information.

(b) SUBJECTS FOR RECOMMENDATIONS.—The recommendations under subsection (a) shall address at least the following:

(1) The rights that an individual who is a subject of individually identifiable health information should have.

(2) The procedures that should be established for the exercise of such rights.

(3) The uses and disclosures of such information that should be authorized or required.

(c) REGULATIONS.—

(1) IN GENERAL.—If legislation governing standards with respect to the privacy of individually identifiable health information transmitted in connection with the transactions described in section 1173(a) of the Social Security Act (as added by section 262) is not enacted by the date that is 36 months after the date of the enactment of this Act, the Secretary of Health and Human Services shall promulgate final regulations containing such standards not later than the date that is 42 months after the date of the enactment of this Act. Such regulations shall address at least the subjects described in subsection (b).

(2) PREEMPTION.—A regulation promulgated under paragraph (1) shall not supercede [sic] a contrary provision of State law, if the provision of State law imposes requirements, standards, or implementation specifications that are more

stringent than the requirements, standards, or implementation specifications imposed under the regulation.

(d) CONSULTATION.—In carrying out this section, the Secretary of Health and Human Services shall consult with—

(1) the National Committee on Vital and Health Statistics established under section 306(k) of the Public Health Service Act (42 U.S.C. 242k(k)); and

(2) the Attorney General.

APPENDIX
E

Committee Biographies

Paul D. Clayton (chair) is a professor of medical informatics (in medicine and radiology) and chair of the Department of Medical Informatics at Columbia University. He is also director of the clinical information services department at Columbia-Presbyterian Medical Center in the City of New York. After receiving a Ph.D. in physics from the University of Arizona, Dr. Clayton spent 15 years as part of the medical informatics group at the University of Utah and LDS Hospital in Salt Lake City, Utah. His current research interests are in the areas of medical information visualization, simplification of user interfaces for physician information input, and security and confidentiality of patient data. Dr. Clayton led the Columbia Presbyterian Medical Center (CPMC) initiative to implement an Integrated Advanced Information Management System that provides access to clinical information for CPMC health care providers, faculty, and students. Dr. Clayton has served on the editorial boards of several journals and is president-elect of the American Medical Informatics Association. He is an elected fellow of the American College of Medical Informatics and the Institute of Medicine.

W. Earl Boebert is with Sandia National Laboratories. Prior to joining Sandia, he was the founder and chief scientist of Secure Computing Technology Corporation (SCTC), predecessor to Secure Computing Corporation (SCC). At SCTC/SCC he led the development of the LOCK, Secure Network Server, and Sidewinder systems. He has 35 years of experience in the computer industry, with more than 20 of them in computer security

247

and cryptography. He is the holder of three and coholder of four patents in the field, is author and coauthor of a book and numerous papers, and has lectured widely. He has been a member of numerous government and industry working groups and panels in the United States and Canada, including the System Security Study Committee of the National Research Council, which produced the report *Computers at Risk*.

Gordon H. DeFriese is professor of social medicine, epidemiology, and health policy and administration at the University of North Carolina at Chapel Hill. He received a B.S. (sociology and political science, 1963) from Middle Tennessee State University, an M.S. (sociology, 1966) from the University of Kentucky, and a Ph.D. (medical sociology, 1967) from the University of Kentucky College of Medicine. He has served as director of the Cecil G. Sheps Center for Health Services Research since 1973. He previously served as director of the North Carolina Cooperative Health Information System and has served on various subcommittees of the U.S. National Committee on Vital and Health Statistics. Dr. DeFriese has served on numerous state and national committees related to health care, primarily in the fields of health care policy and prevention, and he is a member of the Institute of Medicine.

Susan P. Dowell is executive vice president and chief operating officer for Medicus Systems Corporation. She received a B.S. (medical record administration, 1974) from Daemen College and an M.B.A. (1986) from the University of Seattle. Ms. Dowell's position with Medicus involves her with industry associations, including the American Health Information Management Association, of which she served, among other positions, as president; the Illinois Health Information Management Association, at which she was project manager for HL-7;[1] and the Washington State Health Information Management Association, where she served as president and coeditor of the state newsletter. She is also a member of the medical record committee of the Center for Healthcare Information Management and a member of the Healthcare Information Management and Systems Society, the Healthcare Financial Management Association, and the National Association of Healthcare Quality. Ms. Dowell speaks frequently on computer-based patient record strategies, data quality, clinical data systems, quality assurance, productivity and performance standards, information systems strategies, and managed care strategies. She has also

---

[1]HL-7 is a specification for a health data-interchange standard designed to facilitate the transfer of health data resident on different and disparate computer systems in a health care setting.

published numerous articles in the *Journal for the American Health Informa-* *tion Management Association, Topics in Health Information Management,* and *Computers in Healthcare.*

Mary L. Fennell received a Ph.D. in sociology from Stanford University, specializing in the application of organization theory to health care organizations. She has held academic positions at the University of Illinois at Chicago and the Pennsylvania State University. She is currently professor of sociology and community health at Brown University, where she is also affiliated with the Center on Gerontology and Health Care Research. Dr. Fennell teaches courses on health policy, health professions and organizations, organizational theory, and research methods in organizations.

Dr. Fennell is best known for her work on *Diffusion of Medical Innovation* (with Richard Warnecke, published by Plenum in 1988) and for a series of articles on multihospital system structure and governance (with Jeffrey Alexander), which have appeared in the *Administrative Science Quarterly,* the *Journal of Health and Social Behavior,* the *Academy of Management Journal,* and *Medical Care Review.* She has recently published papers on organizational change in the U.S. health care sector and on the changing organizational context of professional work (in the *Annual Review of Sociology* and the *Journal of Health and Social Behavior*). She is currently working on a manuscript (with Kevin Leicht) that will examine recent changes in managerial work and professional practice across the fields of medicine, law, science, and engineering.

Dr. Fennell has led or collaborated on more than a dozen externally funded research projects in the areas of organizational change in health care, innovation diffusion, professional careers, and interorganizational linkage and alliance formation among health care organizations. She is currently studying the development of linkages between acute care and long-term care providers in rural areas and the dissemination of clinical practice innovation in changing health care organizations.

Dr. Fennell served as the editor of the *Journal of Health and Social Behavior* from 1990 through 1993 and has served on advisory or review committees for the Agency for Health Care Policy Research and the Robert Wood Johnson Foundation. She is active in the American Sociological Association, the Association for Health Services Research, the Academy of Management, and the Gerontological Society of America.

Kathleen A. Frawley is vice-president of legislative and public policy services for the American Health Information Management Association. In this position, she provides advocacy at the federal level and testifies before Congress and federal agencies on issues affecting health information management professionals. She previously worked at the Jamaica

Hospital Medical Center in New York, where she served as director of medical records, administrator of medical information systems, and vice president and counsel. From 1976 to 1981, she served as chief of medical record services for the U.S. Public Health Service in New York, and for two years prior to that as the director of the Missouri Hospital Discharge System. Ms. Frawley holds a law degree from New York Law School, an M.S. in health services administration from Wagner College, and a certificate in health record administration. She has lectured and published widely on health information management and confidentiality issues and is a member of several professional organizations. She currently cochairs the work group on confidentiality, privacy, and security for the Computer-based Patient Record Institute. Ms. Frawley was appointed in July 1996 by the Secretary of Health and Human Services to a four-year term on the National Committee on Vital and Health Statistics.

John Glaser is vice president and chief information officer for Partners Healthcare System. He was founding chair of the College of Healthcare Information Management Executives, is past president of the Healthcare Information Management Systems Society, and was the 1994 recipient of the John Gall award for health care chief information officer of the year. Dr. Glaser previously managed the health care information systems consulting practice at Arthur D. Little. He is the author of more than 40 publications on health information systems and holds a Ph.D. (health care information systems) from the University of Minnesota.

Richard A. Kemmerer is professor and chair of the computer science department at the University of California at Santa Barbara. He is a nationally known consultant in computer security and formal verification. He has written widely on computer security, formal specification and verification, software testing, programming languages, and software complexity measures. Dr. Kemmerer received a B.S. (mathematics, 1961) from Pennsylvania State University and an M.S. (computer science, 1976) and a Ph.D. (computer science, 1979) from the University of California at Los Angeles. He is a fellow of the IEEE Computer Society and a member of the Association for Computing Machinery (ACM), the International Federation for Information Processing Working Group 11.3 on Database Security, and the International Association for Cryptologic Research. He is also the past chair of the IEEE Technical Committee on Security and Privacy and a past member of the advisory board for the ACM's Special Interest Group on Security, Audit, and Control. He served on the National Bureau of Standards' Computer and Telecommunications Security Council and on the NRC's study committee that produced *Computers at Risk*. Dr. Kemmerer has served on the editorial boards of the *IEEE Trans-*

actions on Software Engineering and the *ACM Computing Surveys*, and he is currently editor-in-chief of the *IEEE Transactions on Software Engineering*.

Carl E. Landwehr heads the Computer Security Section of the Center for High Assurance Computer Systems at the U.S. Naval Research Laboratory. He has led a variety of research projects to advance technologies for computer security and high-assurance systems and has served on review panels for high-assurance research and development programs at the National Aeronautics and Space Administration and the National Security Agency. Dr. Landwehr chairs an international defense panel on secure information systems and serves as an expert consultant to the North Atlantic Treaty Organization. The International Federation for Information Processing (IFIP) awarded him its Silver Core for his work as founding chair of IFIP Working Group 11.3 on database security, and the IEEE Computer Society awarded him its Golden Core for his work on behalf of its Technical Committee on Security and Privacy. He has served on the editorial boards of the *High Integrity Systems Journal, IEEE Transactions on Software Engineering,* and the *Journal of Computer Security.* He received a B.S. (engineering, 1968) from Yale University, an M.S. (computer and communication sciences, 1970) from the University of Michigan, and a Ph.D. (computer and communication sciences, 1974) from the University of Michigan.

Thomas C. Rindfleisch is director of the Center for Advanced Medical Informatics at the Stanford University School of Medicine. He received a B.S. (physics, 1962) from Purdue University and an M.S. (physics, 1965) from the California Institute of Technology. For more than 20 years, Mr. Rindfleisch has developed open, network-based, distributed computing resources for biomedical informatics applications, first on the ARPANET and subsequently on the Internet. Mr. Rindfleisch leads a team whose ongoing research includes context-based information retrieval and management, multimedia distributed intelligent e-mail systems, mobile pen-based computing systems, information management and access architectures, and security architectures. His interest in privacy and security issues has grown out of real-world experiences in developing and managing nationally networked computing resources. He is a member of the National Library of Medicine Biomedical Library Review Committee and the Federal Networking Council Advisory Committee, a fellow of the American College of Medical Informatics, and a member of the American Association for Artificial Intelligence. He has served on numerous government committees examining information technology applications to health care and on Stanford University advisory committees for information architecture design and implementation strategies.

Sheila A. Ryan received a Ph.D. from the University of Arizona and has held positions as assistant professor, acting dean, associate professor, and dean of nursing at Creighton University in Omaha, Nebraska. At present, she is dean and professor at the School of Nursing and director of Medical Center Nursing at the University of Rochester. Dr. Ryan has developed and conducted numerous funded research projects and has published extensively in books and journals about faculty practice, computer systems, and future models of alternative delivery systems; she has lectured and consulted nationally and internationally. Dr. Ryan serves on many boards of directors of community and health-related organizations locally, regionally, and nationally. She is considered one of the nursing profession's national orators. Dr. Ryan is a fellow of the American Academy of Nursing, program director of the Commonwealth Fund Executive Nurse Fellowship Program, and treasurer of the National League for Nursing. She is also a member of the Institute of Medicine.

Bruce J. Sams, Jr., received a B.A. (1951) from the Georgia Institute of Technology and an M.D. (1955) from Harvard Medical School. He received postgraduate training in internal medicine and hematology at the University of North Carolina, Chapel Hill; the University of California, San Francisco; and the Massachusetts General Hospital. Dr. Sams was a member of the Permanente Medical Group (TPMG) in Northern California from 1963 to 1993 and served as executive director of the group from 1976 to 1991. He retired from TPMG in 1993 and does private consulting. He is a fellow of the American College of Physicians, a distinguished fellow of the American College of Physician Executives, and a member of the Institute of Medicine.

Peter Szolovits is head of the Clinical Decision-Making Group in the Massachusetts Institute of Technology (MIT) Laboratory for Computer Science and a professor of computer science and engineering at MIT, where he teaches classes in artificial intelligence (AI), computer languages, knowledge-based application systems, and medical information science. Dr. Szolovits received B.S. (physics, 1970) and Ph.D. (information science, 1974) degrees from the California Institute of Technology. His research centers on the application of AI methods to problems of medical decision making. He has worked on problems of diagnosis, therapy planning, execution, and monitoring for various medical conditions, as well as on computational aspects of genetic counseling. Dr. Szolovits was editor of the first volume to summarize medical AI work in 1982. His interests in AI include knowledge representation, qualitative reasoning, and probabilistic inference. Dr. Szolovits has published extensively and is on the editorial board of several journals, was program cochairman of the 1992

National Conference on AI, and has been a founder of and consultant for numerous companies that apply AI to problems of commercial interest. He is a fellow of the American Association for Artificial Intelligence and of the American College of Medical Informatics.

Robbie G. Trussell is the senior project manager of pharmacy systems for the Presbyterian Healthcare System based in Dallas, Texas. She received a B.S. (pharmacy, 1972) from the University of Mississippi. She serves as a clinical faculty practitioner for the University of Texas School of Pharmacy. Her areas of expertise include clinical information systems, clinical decision support, systems integration, systems implementation, and pharmacy automation. She is considered one of the pharmacy industry's experts in automation. Ms. Trussell is a fellow of the Healthcare Information and Management Systems Society and currently serves on the board of directors for the organization. She is also a fellow of the American Society of Health-System Pharmacists. She has presented numerous papers relating to automation in pharmacy.

Elizabeth Ward has worked for 23 years in health care, specializing in community health and community mental health services. For half of that time she has been involved in the development of health information systems ranging from automated medical records to large data systems to be used for surveillance and other research activities. Ms. Ward graduated from the University of Washington in 1968 with an M.S. in nursing. Prior to working in Washington, she was Director of Public Health in Alaska. She is currently Assistant Secretary of Epidemiology, Health Statistics, and Public Health Laboratories for the Washington State Department of Health. Ms. Ward has recently been appointed to the National Committee for Vital and Health Statistics.

Paul M. Schwartz (special advisor) is a professor of law at the University of Arkansas School of Law. He is a leading international expert in the field of informational privacy who has published and lectured on issues concerning computers and privacy in the United States and Europe. In this country, his articles and essays have appeared in periodicals such as the *Columbia Law Review, Vanderbilt Law Review, Hastings Law Journal, Iowa Law Review, American Journal of Comparative Law*, and the *Partisan Review*. Professor Schwartz has provided advice and testimony to numerous governmental bodies in the United States and Europe. In 1994 he testified regarding the protection of privacy in health care reform before a subcommittee of the U.S. House of Representatives. He has acted as a consultant to a study of transborder data flows sponsored by the Canadian Ministry of Justice and as one of the investigators preparing a formal evaluation of U.S. data protection law for the Commission of the European Union. Professor Schwartz also served as an expert in international privacy law in a recent groundbreaking case before the Texas Supreme Court. Paul Schwartz is a graduate of Yale Law School, where he served as a senior editor of the *Yale Law Journal*. He received his undergraduate education at Brown University.

Index